Making Sense of Portfolios:
a Guide for Nursing Students

Making Sense of Portfolios:
a Guide for Nursing Students

Fiona Timmins

 Open University Press

Open University Press
McGraw-Hill Education
McGraw-Hill House
Shoppenhangers Road
Maidenhead
Berkshire
England
SL6 2QL

email: enquiries@openup.co.uk
world wide web: www.openup.co.uk

and Two Penn Plaza, New York, NY 10121-2289, USA

First published 2008

A catalogue record of this book is available from the British Library

ISBN-13: 978-0-335-22257-5 (pb)   978-0-335-22258-2 (hb)
ISBN-10: 0-335-22257-9 (pb)   0-335-22258-7 (hb)

Library of Congress Cataloging-in-Publication Data
CIP data applied for

Typeset by RefineCatch Limited, Bungay, Suffolk
Printed in Great Britain by Bell and Bain Ltd, Glasgow

The *McGraw·Hill* Companies

Contents

List of tables, figures and boxes

Tables

Figures

Boxes

1

Learning in the Context of the Portfolio

Fiona Timmins

Introduction • How do people learn? • Adult learning • Identifying learning needs • Learning from experience • Conclusion • Summary of key points • Recommended further reading • References

Introduction

Many Schools of Nursing use a portfolio as a method of both formative and summative assessment (Rassin *et al.* 2006). So you may have come across portfolios that you complete as a component of a programme that is awarded a mark (summative) or not (formative). A portfolio is a collection and cohesive account of work-based learning that contains relevant evidence from practice and critical reflection on this evidence. Its primary purpose is to display achievement of your learning and knowledge development. Most commonly the portfolio is a hand-held document, such as a ring binder, that you, as a student, carry with you to prepare and complete while you are actually gaining your practical clinical experience within the clinical practice environment; it can also be in electronic format. You will learn more specific details about portfolios as the book progresses, but for now we will consider one underlying principle: self-directed learning. While an important underpinning concept within portfolio use is its firm entrenchment in learning from nursing practice experience (Hull *et al.* 2005), equally important is the fact that this learning is usually self-directed. This means that you take responsibility for completing the portfolio and there is relative freedom with task completion, often with minimal direction and guidelines. This can ultimately result in difficulties, wherein you as a student may struggle to understand what exactly is expected from you, or you may receive conflicting direction when you seek advice, which can occur in the absence of detailed guidelines. You may not be exactly sure how to put your practice experiences into the portfolio folder, or how you could organize them or link them together. While some Schools develop quite detailed guidelines, you may also experience the opposite.

Remember!

Portfolios that you are expected to complete as a component of a nursing programme may be awarded a mark/grade (summative assessment) or not (formative assessment).

While you are expected to complete the portfolio in this self-directed way, you may feel that you have received insufficient guidance by way of documentation or in the classroom. While this is a source of confusion and frustration for many students, and indeed you may even question a Nursing School's seemingly lax approach in this matter, it is important to understand that the thinking behind a minimalist intervention is firmly rooted in one philosophy of adult education – self-directed learning. This is often referred to as *andragogy*, and suggests adults are quite capable of independent learning and that, unlike young children, they do not need to be told everything that they need to know (Knowles *et al.* 1998). We need, therefore, to consider your learning as a nursing student, within the portfolio, in light of this.

Activity 1

To what extent are you able to learn independently?

Have you ever learned a topic or skill totally by yourself?

How did you do this?

Have you ever learned a topic or skill partially independently or did you require instruction?

If so, what type of instruction did you require?

You may write down your thoughts on this before proceeding with the chapter.

Although self-directed learning is but one approach to teaching, a unified theory of adult education does not exist. For several decades now the whole notion of how people learn has been explored by academics interested in the field of adult education. Although several theories are proposed, no one theory exists that is sufficient to explain all the complexity of the teaching and learning process. Several theories of both cognitive and behaviourist orientation are posited (Quinn 2000) to underpin a variety of teaching approaches within nurse education, with no one theory emerging as sufficient to explain the range of human behaviours involved in the learning situation. There is agreement, however, that within university education students ought not to be passive recipients of knowledge but, rather, actively involved in attaining their own learning goals (McCauley and McClelland 2004). Although passive learning by students in university during lectures is commonplace, many agree that at least some learning at this level should be of a self-directed nature, thus conducted independently (Quinn 2000; McCauley and McClelland 2004). The advantages of the lecture method include a proven track record of success over a number of years within the university system and its efficient use of resources (Quinn 2000). Within nurse education lecturing is appropriate for teaching broad concepts related to a topic and describing new and unusual situations, but as familiarity with subjects develops nurse educators hold the view that nursing students ought to be increasingly self-directed (Quinn 2000). Applying this belief to portfolio use, nursing students provided with a range of lectures on a variety of aspects of nursing and subsequently immersed in clinical experience are often expected independently to put this prior learning together in portfolio format, to demonstrate their ability to apply their initial learning. This chapter is concerned with understanding the fundamentals of how people learn in this self-directed way.

Activity 2

Think about your last experience at a lecture or being taught in the classroom. To what extent were you actively involved in learning?

Would you describe your learning from this lecture as substantial? Can you recall what you learned?

Think about a project that you had to complete on your own at some time. To what extent were you actively involved in learning?

Would you describe your learning from this project as substantial? Can you recall what you learned?

Write down your thoughts on this before proceeding with the chapter.

How do people learn?

Self-direction indicates that many adults can learn independently in certain areas, without the need for formalized tuition. Self-direction is a universal human attribute that most people possess to some extent (Guglielmino *et al.* 2004). Interest in self-directed learning within education lies in a 40-year tradition of research and writing in the field of adult self-directed learning, stemming from the United States of America (USA), Canada and the United Kingdom (UK) (Guglielmino *et al.* 2004). This research is described as 'one of the most active streams of inquiry in adult education in the US in the last 40 years' (Guglielmino *et al.* 2004: 11). This interest in the area is also reflected in recent literature in nurse education. You will see from these statements that independent learning by adults is an accepted and widely researched phenomenon. Nurse educators' interest in this as a teaching and learning method has increased over the past 20 years, and its principles are applied in many areas including portfolio use.

There is an interesting historical analysis of the development of self-direction in the USA in Guglielmino *et al.* (2004). In this paper the development of self-direction is traced back to early colonial America whereby education of self was commonplace and indeed essential to survival (Guglielmino *et al.* 2004). Early research in the area indicated that self-directed learning was common in the USA in the seventeenth century and was associated with reading and literacy. In the eighteenth century, borrowers who could afford to do so read extensively from subscription libraries, and this later expanded to a wider community with the development of public libraries in the nineteenth and twentieth centuries (Knowles 1962). Thus the library was a large support in the self-direction movement (Guglielmino *et al.* 2004).

Activity 3

Interestingly, during this period people were deprived of learning resources for economic and other reasons. Literacy itself was a barrier to learning. When barriers were broken down, for instance when access to public libraries increased, people jumped at the chance to become self-educated.

Compare this to your situation now, and describe your motivation and enthusiasm for learning.

A trend towards research and writing in the area of self-direction thus developed in the USA in the 1960s. Carl Rogers's (1969) seminal work was central to this (Guglielmino *et al.* 2004). Knowles (Knowles 1962, 1970, 1989; Knowles *et al.* 1998) was also a key writer in this field. Although nurse education does not profess to hold a specific theory of education, theories that espouse self-direction such as Rogers's and Knowles's work have been highly influential in nurse education in the UK and elsewhere (Quinn 2000).

Merriam (1987: 88) suggests that:

> a theory of adult learning would be a set of inter-related principles that enable us to understand how adults learn. Carried a step further, if we understand how adults learn we should be able to predict when and how learning will take place, and . . . arrange for its occurrence.

From the perspective of the self-direction movement, adults are inherently capable of self-directed learning, and this occurrence can be traced back several hundred years. Given the extent of research in this area and its relative popularity within nurse education settings, nurse educators consider it is a useful framework within which to consider learners that attend nurse education programmes. Whether it is using public libraries, or reading newspapers, adults have the capacity to be self-taught to a certain extent. This is not suggesting the abandonment of the university and education system as we know it, but rather, as Merriam (1987) outlines, provides us with an understanding of learning that can enable educators to capture and encourage and maximize learning in this way.

Portfolios, the theme of this book, which will be discussed in more detail in later chapters, are primarily based on this notion of self-direction and individualized student learning (Garrett and Jackson 2006). Several authors are in agreement that self-direction is a fundamental principle of adult learning that is integral to the portfolio. Furthermore, where writers allude to a theory supporting portfolio use in nursing it is usually either Knowles or Rogers who are suggested as rationales or supporting frameworks (Jasper 1995; Spence and El-Ansari 2004). Thus portfolio use within nurse education is ultimately associated with the ability of adults to engage in self-directed learning. It is acknowledged, for example, that qualified nurses are capable of being self-directed with regard to maintaining professional development. The aim of portfolio use in this group is to encourage and quantify this self-directed learning so that private learning may become public, thus making it available to viewing by others. Similarly, undergraduate nursing students will undoubtedly seek out new information and make personal observations of learning during the programme, and portfolio use aims to provide a valid and reliable way of structuring these observations and maximizing the learning from this. Before proceeding to discuss the portfolio in more detail it is worth considering the principles of self-directed adult learning in more detail, and in particular its emphasis and place within contemporary nurse education. Knowles and Rogers are frequently cited in texts and papers in the field of nursing. Both theories will now be briefly described to provide further exposition of the way in which adults learn in the educational context.

Adult learning

Rogers's (1969, 1983) writings heralded the foundation of humanistic theory and yielded a consideration of the individualistic nature of learning. Rather than a broad assumption that all individuals learn in a similar manner, academics began to consider that, for teaching to be successful, individual human factors need consideration. Thus the notion of individual motivation to learn such as self-concept and self-esteem became popular. Rogers suggests that rather than acting as authority figures, educators should *facilitate* learning through the understanding, acknowledgement and consideration of unique motivations. Student-centred learning approaches are emphasized. This involves the creation of environments that emphasize freedom for individual development and, according to Rogers (1969, 1983), enable students to become more adaptable and self-directed. Contemporary texts encourage nurse educators to use this approach (Quinn 2000) and it is one that nursing students favour (Harvey and Vaughan 1990).

Activity 4

Think back to Activity 1, and any instruction that you may have required for an activity. List the important elements.

Now think back to when you learned to ride a bicycle (or tricycle); or think of a situation when you may have observed this learning activity. In most cases 'prompts' were given to the person, rather than a detailed explanation of every aspect of riding. The relevant equipment was provided, the roadway was sufficient for the task, and those assisting were encouraging and supportive. Write down your thoughts on this.

It is these elements (environment and support) that are key to Rogers's theory of facilitation that encourages self-directed learning. Outline to what extent you agree with this notion.

Rogers (1969, 1983) explicates empathy, congruence and positive regard as necessary conditions for facilitation. Rogers (1983) also emphasizes the importance of the facilitator being genuine. Facilitation as a concept that relates to how adults learn has been enthusiastically employed by nurse education for a number of years. Small student numbers at hospital-based Schools of Nursing were especially suitable for this facilitative method (Quinn 2000). Although this is less common with the advent of university education and inherent large class sizes, nurse educators retain a commitment to facilitative student-centred methods, favouring these as a method of achieving adult learning.

A concept analysis (Burrows 1997) of the term facilitation arising from the work of Rogers (1969, 1983) is revealing. Emerging critical attributes are identified as: genuine mutual respect; the development of a partnership in learning; a dynamic goal-orientated process; the practice of critical reflection (Burrows 1997). In order for facilitation to take place in the learning situation all of these factors need to be present. Therefore, although self-directed learning in this context is student-led, it requires the support of the teacher, as facilitator of learning. This facilitation, though, is not a directive process but rather a helping relationship where there is genuineness, respect and partnership, with both working towards set goals. Burrows (1997: 396) further redefines facilitation as 'a goal-orientated dynamic process, in which participants work together in an atmosphere of genuine mutual respect, in order to learn through critical reflection'. The consequences of facilitation are that students become active, enthusiastic, self-directed learners; the facilitator becomes a co-learner and relinquishes control. Students gain control and learning goals are achieved. You may begin to understand that the direction that you may require in portfolio preparation is a great deal more subtle and less sophisticated than you had imagined. Perhaps initial schooling and university education have been quite directive for students and developing independent learning skills are thus more challenging. The support for independent learning, as suggested by Rogers, is the environment and warmth and genuineness of relationships that one encounters in the learning experience. Clinical staffs are therefore pivotal in supporting you with your portfolio; however, this does not necessarily mean that they direct you, but rather that they support and encourage you to find your own way, just like riding a bicycle in Activity 4.

Activity 5

Think of a person that you have worked closely with in the clinical area.

List the important elements of your relationship with that person.

Did these elements support your learning? Write down the ways in which they may have supported you.

Do any of your ideas concur with Rogers's ideas?

Rogers's humanistic theory (1969, 1983) enjoys popularity in nurse education settings. Similarly, Knowles's (1962, 1970, 1989; Knowles *et al.* 1998) theory of andragogy enjoys success. In this model Knowles also refers to the teacher as a facilitator, but focuses more on the conditions necessary within the person for learning to take place. Knowles advocates the use of the term andragogy to describe the art and science of helping adults to learn. Andragogy is an 'organized and sustained effort to assist adults to learn in a way that enhances their capacity to function as self-directed learners' (Mezirow 1983: 136). Knowles initially proposed andragogy as the opposite of *pedagogy*, the manner in which children learn, thus suggesting a dichotomy between the two. However, he later acknowledged that this dichotomy was not so extreme, and that at times both pedagogy and andragogy may be appropriate to adults, depending on their given circumstances.

Knowles identifies four key components of adult learning: self-concept, past experience, readiness to learn and the diagnosis of learning needs. It is believed that once we understand how adults learn we should be able to predict when and how best learning will take place (Merriam 1987). The andragogical approach suggests that learners are self-directed and draw on their own personal experience (Howard 1993). Knowles also suggests that self-concept influences adult self-directed learning. *Self-concept* refers to adult learners having a concept of being responsible for their own decisions (Knowles 1989). The more adult learners are involved in the planning of their own learning, the more likely it is that their goals will be attained. Learners' self-concept assumes that adults have a perception of being responsible for their own decisions and their own lives. Once adults have this perception they develop a need to be treated by others as being capable of self-direction. Knowles contends that when adults discover this perception they resist and resent situations in which they feel others are imposing their will on them. However, facilitators can work to create learning experiences in which adults are helped to maintain their transition to self-directing learners.

This theory emphasizes, like humanism, the individual nature of learning. Knowles contends that adult learners volunteer themselves for their education to achieve their personal goals. Due to this they are motivated, orientated towards learning, thus enthusiastic, self-directing and ready to embark upon the relevant learning. This will seem certainly relevant for nursing students like you, who have chosen nursing as a career. Knowles suggests that adults are capable of being self-directed in their own learning and can diagnose their own learning needs. Adults can identify what it is they need to know in a given situation

This may at first seem a strange concept for you to grapple with within a nurse education programme, where surely essential aspects of the profession need to be taught directly to students. However, as Knowles suggests, a purely pedagogical approach simply provides the relevant direction with little consideration of you as a student having a proactive place in the learning situation. From Knowles's perspective, to an extent, pedagogy excludes self-direction in learning. Andragogy, on the other hand, accepts the need for a pedagogical approach but also recognizes that within adults there are certain conditions that make the adult capable of independent learning and that these can be maximized within learning situations.

Knowles's view on learning is particularly useful for you as a nursing student to understand how you may learn as you progress through a variety of learning situations in your clinical practice rotations. While each student may have received the relevant information in class about the relevant patient conditions, each clinical experience carries with it specific learning objectives.

Furthermore, each situation is quite different and you as a student are quite different to everyone else. You may come to the situation with your own previous experience that may alter your learning outcomes. For example, you may have previously displayed great strengths in relation to communication, but require more experience with planning care. Therefore the learning needs in the situation, while still remaining within set learning objectives for the experience, can potentially be adapted to fit in more with your prior experience, learning needs and readiness to learn.

These are core principles of Knowles's theory of andragogy. It is worth noting, however, that while self-direction has been described as being a fully independent activity in some previous studies on the topic, it is generally accepted that this level of independence varies between individuals and that in a formalized education system such as nurse education, learners need to be supported to achieve this self-direction (Knowles *et al.* 1998). Quite simply, self-direction within nursing does not imply being given a reading list, or quiet time away from the clinical nursing environment in which to read; it occurs within the context of a facilitative relationship and clear parameters. This can become more formalized through the use of learning contracts or portfolio, thus allowing learning to be evidenced and used as a scaffold to support future learning. It can also permit self-direction in learning to be submitted for formal assessment and be assigned a grade within an educational programme.

Thus what is primarily an independent activity occurs within the structure of a facilitative relationship, with appropriate guidelines. The result for each student is quite different and unique depending on individual experiences, goals, readiness and motivation. It is important, however, for Nursing Schools to recognize that students may need to be guided by the teacher on how to undertake effective self-directive learning (Milligan 1995). An assumption ought not to be made that adults are automatically independent learners (Knowles *et al.* 1998). Indeed, particular types of first- and second-level schooling could render some students quite dependent upon teacher direction (Hartree 1984). Physics students' ability to be self-directed has been examined (McCauley and McClelland 2004). The findings revealed that many of the students were not yet ready to be self-directed and higher achievers were more likely to be self-directed. These students were not 'well prepared to self-direct in their own learning'. However, for those students without self-directed 'tendencies', the portfolio can 'help to nurture and develop them, given a facilitative climate' (Joyce 2005: 458).

While there are benefits to attempting to maximize the self-directed learning ability of adults within nurse education programmes, there are of course many challenges. Where self-direction is encouraged through portfolio use, for example, some students may lack motivation, and in the absence of formalized assessment may fail to produce the necessary work. Furthermore, where portfolios are submitted for assessment there can be difficulty assigning a grade to what are very unique and individual pieces of work. In addition, as previously pointed out, students may not yet be ready for self-directed learning (McCauley and McClelland 2004). These challenges will be discussed in more detail in later chapters, but for the moment further consideration of the conditions for adult learning is required.

Activity 6

Think back to your first formal teaching class in the course that you are attending. What prior knowledge or experience influenced how you received this information?

Think back to your visit or placement to an area of nursing practice.

What prior knowledge or experience did you have about the area, clients or their conditions? Write down your responses.

You will see from your responses above that, just as Knowles suggests, adults take significant past experience to learning situations. Whether this influence is very small, and just leaves us with an inkling of what the class topic may be about, or whether it is more substantial (perhaps you have worked on the ward area as a nursing auxiliary or nurse assistant), your previous experience can be influential. *Past experience* has a significant impact on adult learning (Knowles 1989). It can influence perception of events. This assumption implies that adults enter education with a greater volume and a different quality of experiences from that of children. Knowles (1989) suggests that, due to this, adults can learn from other adults in the group, hence the value of group discussion. However, Knowles does contend that previous experiences can also achieve negative affects. Biases and preconceived ideas may be a barrier to new ideas and fresh perceptions.

Activity 7

Identify a learning situation (in your life in general) where your own previous experience was beneficial.

Identify a learning situation (in your life in general) where your own previous experience created preconceived ideas for you.

Write down your responses.

From the above examples you can identify, as Knowles has outlined, that there are both positive and negative consequences of previous experience. However, previous experience simply cannot be extinguished; what is required in the utilization of self-directed learning methods is an acknowledgement of these experiences, and continued awareness of their influence. Acknowledging these at the outset of self-directed learning can be helpful. This is often the first phase of self-directed learning contracts, and serves to inform and perhaps modify learning goals. The role of previous experience is not usually specifically referred to when a portfolio is being prepared by undergraduate nursing students. Qualified nurses may cite their previous nursing experiences and courses undertaken as part of their professional portfolio to highlight their own personal and professional development. Rather than focusing specifically on past professional experience, as is the case with qualified nurses' portfolios, aspects of students' past experiences are drawn out through the use of reflection, which will be discussed in more detail in Chapter 3. Through the use of models of reflection, a student's past experience may be exposed and perhaps its ultimate effect upon learning realized. Models of reflection usually require a personal description of some events and one's reactions. These are inherently personal and based in prior experience. Thus the self-directed learning situation is ultimately influenced by past experience. Indeed, the andragogical approach to learning encourages learners to draw on their experience (Howard 1993).

Knowles also places emphasis on adults' individual *readiness to learn* – this assumption suggests that adults become ready to learn what they need to know when they recognize a gap or learning need exists. The effectiveness of teaching methods can be reduced if a student is not *ready to learn* (Knowles 1989). The internal motivation of adult learners is an important factor in this readiness. If, as with many adult learners, students are on a chosen course such as nursing, internal motivation is presumably high. However, if the motivation to learn is coming from an external source, for example an employer requires course attendance but there is little personal motivation, then a person may not feel ready to learn the particular topic and perhaps learn less than if personal internal motivation existed (Knowles 1989). While readiness to learn is likely to vary within a group of students, it can also vary within individuals depending upon circumstances. Therefore within a classroom situation readiness to learn is not unanimous among the student group and ultimately the extent of maximum learning will vary. Self-directed learning on the other hand can be timed to coincide with readiness. Knowles (1989) contends that it is not necessary to sit by passively and wait for readiness to develop naturally. Readiness can be encouraged through facilitation (as outlined by Rogers earlier in the chapter). The use of a student portfolio provides opportunities for this facilitative relationship to develop. This facilitative climate has proved successful for portfolio production and completion (Joyce 2005). If you as a student can develop your portfolio in your own time, this would obviously allow you to complete it exactly when you feel ready. However, there are obviously difficulties with applying adult learning concepts in this way. This free approach may encourage some students to procrastinate and put the portfolio off. Additionally within the confines of university, for assessment purposes, completion dates are ordinarily required.

Interestingly, researchers have examined students' readiness to learn, notably Guglielmino (1977) and more recently Fisher *et al.* (2001). Fisher *et al.* suggest that their research instrument has increased validity and reliability compared with others. They outline three main factors that they associate with student readiness to become self-directed: self-management, desire for learning and self-control. These overarching categories and their sub-elements are displayed in Table 1.1. Although primarily designed as a research tool, you may be able to identify your strengths and weaknesses in relation to self-directed learning from this table. All of these elements are important to possess in order to engage fully in self-directed learning. By identifying those attributes which you believe you possess and those which you don't you may be able to outline areas that you need to develop in order to become more independent as a learner. This will also give you an outline of the level of responsibility and independence that your tutor or lecturer will expect from you, when you are engaged in a self-directed assessment such as a portfolio.

Knowles (1989) also places great emphasis on the *diagnosis of learning needs* as critical to adult education. It involves the following components: assessment of needs; formulation of objectives; the design of learning experiences and evaluation. As previously mentioned, self-direction may be present in each person to a different extent. It is also dependent upon individual readiness, motivation, orientation towards learning and self-concept. It is also influenced by previous experience. With so many conditions for learning that are independent of the teacher but rather dependent on the learner, it is possible for self-directed efforts to go astray. For many students self-directed learning doesn't take place at all (McCauley and McClelland 2004). Within the portfolio the failure of independent learning can result in students presenting the portfolio with little apparent thought or preparation as a mere collection of items within a folder with no connections between parts (Farrell 2004). This is referred to as the 'shopping trolley' approach (Endacott *et al.* 2004), where literally every component part is just thrown in.

Facilitation is proposed by both Knowles and Rogers as central to supporting student self-direction, and the nurse supervising the student, either as mentor or facilitator, acts as a key person to guide and support the student in this activity (Farrell 2004). While more information will be provided in subsequent chapters with regard to this support and also portfolio structure, it is worth considering the diagnosis of learning needs as central to the portfolio structure. Self-diagnosis of learning needs, that is an individual outlining what it is they need to know, is crucial to the self-direction process (Knowles 1989). Facilitators can also assist with this extrapolation.

As the diagnosis of these needs involves four central components (Table 1.2), these could form an overarching framework to develop a portfolio, given that the very basis for portfolio use stems from the self-direction movement. Diagnosis begins with assessment. Questions could be asked such as those in Box 1.1.

Once these broad personal needs are outlined and merged, if appropriate, with the objectives of the clinical area, or of the particular assessment (some portfolios may have specific objectives), a set of specific objectives for your portfolio may be outlined and included within. This is followed by an outline

Table 1.1 Main factors associated with students' readiness to engage in self-directed learning

Self-management	YES	NO
I manage my time well		
I am self-disciplined		
I am organized		
I set strict time frames		
I have good management skills		
I am methodical		
I am systematic in my learning		
I set specific times for my study		
I solve problems using a plan		
I prioritize my work		
I can be trusted to pursue my own learning		
I prefer to plan my own learning		
I am confident in my ability to search out information		

Desire for learning
I want to learn new information
I enjoy learning new information
I have a need to learn
I enjoy a challenge
I enjoy studying
I critically evaluate new ideas
I like to gather the facts before I make a decision
I like to evaluate what I do
I am open to new ideas
I learn from my mistakes
I need to know why
When presented with a problem I cannot resolve, I will ask for assistance
I often review the way nursing practices are conducted
I need to be in control of what I learn

Self-control
I prefer to set my own goals
I like to make decisions for myself
I am responsible for my own decisions/actions
I am in control of my life
I have high personal standards
I prefer to set my own learning goals
I evaluate my own performance
I am logical
I am responsible
I have high personal expectations
I am able to focus on a problem
I am aware of my own limitations
I can find out information for myself
I have high beliefs in my abilities
I prefer to set my own criteria on which to evaluate my performance

Source: Adapted from Fisher *et al.* (2001).

Table 1.2 Four core components of the diagnosis of learning needs

Assessment of needs
Formulation of objectives
The design of learning experiences
Evaluation

Source: Knowles (1989).

Box 1.1   Questions to prompt diagnosis of learning needs within the portfolio

What is it I need to achieve (from this clinical experience)?

Are there core learning objectives associated with the experience?

Have I particular strengths or weaknesses or previous experiences that I bring to this experience that affect this need?

Are there particular client groups that I am likely to encounter?

Do I have particular interests or motivations around the area that I would like to develop within the portfolio?

---

of the design of the learning experiences that you are going to discuss. Rather than a mix and match of various papers, you are aiming here for a cohesive 'cake mix' approach to your work (Endacott *et al*. 2004), where the parts blend well together.

This means that the various learning experiences that you outline combine together in a meaningful way. The learning experiences could be developed within a framework for reflection, which will be discussed in the next chapter, merging both personal experiences and literature on the topic within. Evaluation according to this model is a key feature in developing the cohesive portfolio. Ask yourself what you have achieved through developing the portfolio? Look back and examine whether you achieved the set learning objectives? And if not, why not?

Remember!

It is always important to self-evaluate your own work.

Identifying learning needs is a popular feature within self-directed learning. Thus it requires more discussion to examine its place within adult learning in general and portfolio use in particular.

Identifying learning needs

Educators have long favoured the 'needs' approach as a means of educating adults (Mason-Attwood and Ellis 1971). Rather than imparting information based on the preferences of administration, or implementing mass programmes designed for general use, this approach attempts to identify and meet the needs of the individual. In a classroom setting this implies that, rather than providing mass lectures that apply to all students, there is an attempt to gain an understanding of the individual needs within the group, or the group learning needs. This can be done simply by the use of a standard questionnaire before onset of a series of lectures, perhaps identifying students' prior experience with the topic and asking them what it is they perceive they need to know. With regard to portfolio use each student is identifying his or her own personal needs, with the support of the facilitator. Unfortunately, providing facilitative support, although optimal, can prove difficult for some areas, as it is a very time-consuming and resource-intensive activity.

Knowles (1989) suggests that assessment of learning needs is critical to adult education. The first step understands what learning needs means. Knowles defines a learning need as the gap between competencies specified and the present level of development by the learner. The crucial element in the assessment of the 'gap' is learners' own perception of the discrepancy between where they are now and where they want to be (Knowles 1989). Educational needs, information needs and learning needs are used interchangeably within the literature. Mason-Attwood and Ellis (1971) suggested that a need is a deficiency that detracts from a person's well-being. These authors described educational needs as those which result from educational deficiency and which can be satisfied by a learning experience.

This striving towards identification and ultimate achievement of learning needs is crucial to the self-direction process (Burrows 1997). Portfolios, while necessarily based around predetermined programme objectives or learning outcomes, require some level of flexibility in terms of permitting students to identify their own learning needs (Pearce 2003). The facilitation of adult learning is ultimately a goal-orientated process (Burrows 1997). Facilitation is also key to the creation of an atmosphere of partnership and respect that positively supports the student. Both of these concepts (identification of learning needs and facilitation) are further key concepts in portfolio development (Glen and Hight 1992). Another concept that is suggested as a crucial attribute of facilitation is critical reflection and this too is a common component in the portfolio process. In addition to self-direction, reflection is the second pillar of portfolio use. Reflection is inherently linked to Knowles's concept of past experience and may also be considered learning through experience (Boud and Walker 1990, 1993). Thus the processes of self-directed learning and facilitation are closely linked to portfolio processes. Another inherent element within many portfolios is learning from experience.

Learning from experience

While the use of reflection within a portfolio has been briefly alluded to and will be further developed in Chapter 3, it is interesting to note that Boud and Walker (1990, 1993) present a new perspective on reflection termed *learning from experience*. Although initially described as a model of reflection designed for students to learn from experience (Boud *et al.* 1985), subsequent ongoing development leads the authors specifically to refer more recently to *workplace learning* (Boud *et al.* 2006). This means that all learning takes place in the context of the working environment and reflection is the means for doing so (Boud and Walker 1990, 1993; Andresen *et al.* 2000; Boud *et al.* 2006). This model of reflection focuses upon work-based learning and thus has particular relevance for nursing student portfolios. It will be described in more detail in Chapter 3.

Nursing students undertake practice placements in a variety of nursing situations. Within these settings, tacit knowledge development is encouraged. Tacit knowledge exists within communities of practice, such as nursing, and is a valuable source of knowledge that can be difficult to recognize or replicate. It consists of 'embodied expertise – a deep understanding of complex, interdependent systems that enables dynamic responses to context-specific problems' (Wenger *et al.* 2002: 9). Tacit knowledge is shared through interaction and informal learning and may be passed directly from one person to the other within the community of practice (Baumard 1999). Knowledge within groups such as nursing is social as well as individual (Wenger *et al.* 2002). Thus knowledge is not necessarily the prerogative of individuals (although they have knowledge); knowledge within communities needs to be shared. Thus a body of knowledge is developed through a 'process of communal involvement' (Wenger *et al.* 2002: 10).

Herbig (Herbig *et al.* 2001: 694) suggests that tacit knowledge among nurses should become more conscious and obvious through the design of 'working structures and processes that give opportunities to reflect upon experiences'. Knowledge is 'not an object that can be stored, owned and moved around like a piece of equipment or a document. It resides in the skills, understandings, and relationships of its members as well as in the tools, documents, and processes that embody aspects of this knowledge' (Wenger *et al.* 2002: 10). For nursing students, tapping into this tacit knowledge represents a challenge. Describing learning experiences within a portfolio approach is one way of drawing this knowledge out. Tacit knowledge is largely acquired from experience, preferably in the environment where the knowledge is required (Sternberg 1999), thus the work-based portfolio is the perfect medium.

In his delineation of knowledge, Baumard (1999) drew upon the work of the Greek philosophers who differentiate between four forms of knowledge:

- *episteme* (abstract generalization);
- *techne* (capability, capacity to accomplish tasks);
- *phronesis* (practical and social wisdom);
- *mètis* (conjectural intelligence).

He described *episteme* as universal knowledge that is shared and general. *Episteme* according to Aristole is knowledge about which we can be certain and it equates to scientific knowledge. *Phronesis* is the opposite: it is personal and meaningful to the individual. It is 'non-scientific, practical, contextual knowledge . . . generated in the intimacy of lived experience' (Baumard 1999: 3). *Techne* is the application of technical knowledge; *mètis* is the combination of explicit and tacit knowledge, the collective and individual and thus the implementation of the four forms of knowledge (Figure 1.1).

From this discussion it is clear that a portfolio, as an exposition of student learning, needs to consider knowledge in its broadest sense. In professional nursing practice portfolios may be used to record nurses' 'embedded practical knowledge' (Melrose 2006). Even though adult learning implies independence in thinking and learning, the evidence within the portfolio ought not to be overtly personal, and rely on *phronesis*, but rather take into account forms of knowledge other than personal. There is an important place for evidence and research even within an interpretive approach to knowledge development (Rolfe and Gardner 2005). Thus inclusion of technical knowledge within the portfolio is important. Similarly, it is important to tap into the wisdom of the

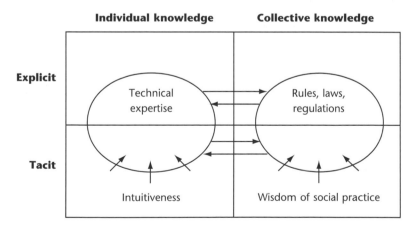

Figure 1.1 Four inseparable types of knowledge (Baumard 1999: 66)

Source: Reproduced by permission of Sage Publications, London, Los Angeles, New Delhi and Singapore. (© Baumard 1999).

nurse in practice, thus gleaning social wisdom. The mechanisms for doing this will be considered in more detail in later chapters.

The portfolio is a vehicle for knowledge development and may aim to display the scholarship of individual students' practice. Riley *et al.* (2002) noted that nursing scholarship has traditionally been viewed as within an academic environment with an emphasis on research within the discipline. Building on Boyer's (1990) work they proposed a new paradigm for defining nursing scholarship. Rather than being solely concerned with the discovery of new knowledge, they suggested other aspects to scholarship: integration and application. In order to document learning, they suggested, based on Boyer (1990), the use of a portfolio supported by evidence and reflection on learning and consideration of implications for future practice. They suggested the portfolio as 'a promising strategy' for the development of this scholarship.

Conclusion

The notion of a reflective portfolio that would allow you as a nursing student to develop and display your scholarship represents a challenge for all those involved. The portfolio primarily originates from the notion that adults are capable of self-directed learning. With this origin acknowledged it is important that key principles of adult learning are incorporated into portfolio use. These are the principles of identification of learning needs, including: assessment of needs; formulation of objectives; the design of learning experiences and evaluation. Within this context there also needs to be acknowledgement and utilization of your previous experience. Facilitation is a key component of self-direction and key personnel need to guide and support you with regard to portfolio use. Self-direction, then, is not solely concerned with learning alone fostered by self-motivation; the help and support of others is useful. Guidelines are also important. The portfolio may have a broad framework of assessment of needs, formulation of objectives, the design of learning experiences and evaluation. It may also consist of multiple entries, where particular learning experiences are outlined and reflected upon. Reflection forms a key component of the learning from experience within a portfolio, and models for this are considered in Chapter 3. Learning from portfolios is ultimately about knowledge development. Baumard's description of knowledge typologies (1999) demonstrates how important it is that the portfolio contains relevant forms of knowledge from a range of sources. What is required within this presentation of knowledge and learning from experience as an adult is a cohesive and comprehensive account of learning. Simply placing a range of articles or other objects in a folder greatly undermines what can be a very important learning tool for you as a student. The purpose of portfolios is considered in more detail in the following chapter.

Summary of key points

* The belief that adults can be self-directed in their own learning is fundamental to the use and development of portfolios within nurse education.
* Self-direction, while new to some students, needs to be supported and encouraged. Facilitation in the clinical area, through developing working relationships, can indirectly assist this process and also pass on the tacit knowledge that students require to build up their portfolio.
* It is important to commence the portfolio by deciding upon your learning needs.
* The portfolio is a testament to your knowledge and learning in the clinical area and ought to be an intelligent account of this, rather than a collection of artefacts.

Recommended further reading

Knowles, M. S. (1989) *The Adult Learner: A Neglected Species*. Houston, TX: Gulf Publishing Company.

Rogers, C. R. (1983) *Freedom to Learn for the 80s*. London: CE Merrill Publishing Company.

Boud, D., Cressey, P. *et al.* (2006) Setting the scene for productive reflection at work, in D. Boud, P. Cressey and P. Doherty (eds) *Productive Reflection at Work*. Oxford: Routledge.

References

Andresen, L., Boud, D., *et al.* (2000) Experience-based learning, in G. Foley (ed.) *Understanding Adult Education and Training*. Sydney: Allen & Unwin.

Baumard, P. (1999) *Tacit Knowledge in Organizations*. London: Sage Publications.

Boud, D., Cressey, P. *et al.* (2006) Setting the scene for productive reflection at work, in D. Boud, P. Cressey and P. Doherty (eds) *Productive Reflection at Work*. Oxford: Routledge.

Boud, D., Keogh, R. *et al.* (1985) Promoting reflection in learning: a model, in D. Boud, D. Walker and R. Keogh (eds), *Reflection: Turning Experience into Learning*. London: Kogan Page.

Boud, D. and Walker, D. (1990) Making the most of experience, *Studies in Continuing Education*, 12(2): 61–80.

Boud, D. and Walker, D. (1993) Barriers to reflection on experience, in D. Boud, R. Cohen and D. Walker (eds), *Using Experience For Learning*. Buckingham: Society for Research into Higher Education and Open University Press.

Boyer, E. L. (1990) *Scholarship Reconsidered: Priorities of the Professorate*. Princeton, NJ: Carnegie Endowment for the Advancement of Teaching.

Burrows, D. E. (1997) Facilitation: a concept analysis, *Journal of Advanced Nursing*, 25(2): 396–404.

Endacott, R., Gray, M. A. *et al.* (2004) Using portfolios in the assessment of learning and competence: the impact of four models, *Nurse Education in Practice*, 4(4): 250–7.

Farrell, M. (2004) Illuminating the essential elements of the competence-based approach to nurse education through an exploration of staff nurses' experiences of its implementation within the practice placement: a phenomenological study. Unpublished Masters thesis, School of Nursing and Midwifery, University College Dublin.

Fisher, M., King, J. *et al.* (2001) Development of a self-directed learning readiness scale for nursing education, *Nurse Education Today*, 21(7): 516–25.

Garrett, B. M. and Jackson, C. (2006) A mobile clinical e-portfolio for nursing and medical students, using wireless personal digital assistants (PDAs), *Nurse Education in Practice*, 6(6): 339–46.

Glen, S. and Hight, N. F. (1992) Portfolios: an 'effective' assessment strategy?, *Nurse Education Today*, 12(6): 416–23.

Guglielmino, J., Long, H. B. *et al.* (2004) Historical perspectives series: self-direction in learning in the United States, *International Journal of Self-Directed Learning*, 1(1): 1–18.

Guglielmino, L. M. (1977) Development of the self-directed learning readiness scale. Unpublished PhD dissertation, University of Georgia.

Hartree, A. (1984) Malcolm Knowles's theory of andragogy: a critique, *International Journal of Lifelong Education*, 3(3): 203–10.

Harvey, T. J. and Vaughan, J. (1990) Student nurse attitudes towards different teaching/learning methods, *Nurse Education Today*, 10(3): 181–5.

Herbig, B., Bussing, A. *et al.* (2001) The role of tacit knowledge in the work context of nursing, *Journal of Advanced Nursing*, 34(5): 687–95.

Howard, S. (1993) Accreditation of prior learning: andragogy in action or a 'cut price' approach to education?, *Journal of Advanced Nursing*, 18: 1817–24.

Hull, C., Redfern, J. *et al.* (2005) *Profiles and Portfolios: A Guide for Health and Social Care*. Basingstoke: Palgrave Macmillan.

Jasper, M. A. (1995) The potential of the professional portfolio for nursing, *Journal of Clinical Nursing*, 15(6): 446–51.

Joyce, P. (2005) A framework for portfolio development in postgraduate nursing practice, *Journal of Clinical Nursing*, 14(4): 456–63.

Knowles, M., Holton, E. *et al.* (1998) *The Adult Learner. The Definitive Classic in Adult Education and Human Resource Development*, 5th edn. Houston, TX: Gulf Publishing.

Knowles, M. S. (1962) *The Adult Education Movement in the United States*. New York: Holt, Rinehart and Winston.

Knowles, M. S. (1970) *The Modern Practice of Adult Education*. New York: Cambridge Books.

Knowles, M. S. (1989) *The Adult learner: A Neglected Species*. Houston, TX: Gulf Publishing Company.

McCauley, V. and McClelland, G. (2004) Further studies in self-directed learning in physics at the University of Limerick, Ireland, *International Journal of Self-Directed Learning*, 1(2): 26–37.

Mason-Attwood, H. and Ellis, J. (1971) The concept of need: an analysis for adult education, *Adult Leadership*, 19: 210–12.

Melrose, S. (2006) Creating a psychiatric mental health portfolio: an assignment activity that works, *Nurse Education in Practice*, 6(5): 288–94.

Merriam, S. B. (1987) Adult learning and theory building: a review, *Adult Education Quarterly*, 37: 187–98.

Mezirow, J. (1983) A critical theory of adult learning and education, in M. Tight (ed.) *Education for Adults: Educational Opportunities for Adults*. Beckenham: Croom Helm in association with the Open University.

Milligan, F. (1995) In defence of andragogy, *Nurse Education Today*, 15(1): 22–7.

Pearce, R. (2003) *Profiles and Portfolios of Evidence*. Cheltenham: Nelson Thornes.

Quinn, F. M. (2000) *The Principles and Practice of Nurse Education*, Cheltenham: Nelson Thornes.

Rassin, M., Silner, D. *et al.* (2006) Departmental portfolio in nursing: an advanced instrument, *Nurse Education in Practice*, 6(1): 55–60.

Riley, J. M., Beal, J. *et al.* (2002) Revisioning nursing scholarship, *Journal of Nursing Scholarship*, 34(4): 383–9.

Rogers, C. R. (1969) *Freedom to Learn*. Columbus, OH: Merrill.

Rogers, C. R. (1983) *Freedom to Learn for the 80s*, London: C. E. Merrill Publishing Company.

Rolfe, G. and Gardner, L. (2005) Towards a nursing science of the unique: evidence, reflexivity and the study of persons, *Journal of Research in Nursing*, 10(3): 297.

Spence, W. and El-Ansari, W. (2004) Portfolio assessment: practice teachers' early experience, *Nurse Education Today*, 24(5): 388–401.

Sternberg, R. J. (1999) What do we know about tacit knowledge? Making the tacit become explicit, in R. J. Sternberg and J. A. Hovarth (eds), *Tacit Knowledge in Professional Practice: Researcher and Practitioner Perspectives*. Mahwah, NJ: Lawrence Erlbaum Associates.

Wenger, E. C., Mc Dermott, R. *et al.* (2002) *Cultivating Communities of Practice: A Guide to Managing Knowledge*. Boston, MA: Harvard Business School Press.

2

The Purpose of Portfolios

Miriam Farrell

Introduction • Defining portfolio • The portfolio as a mechanism for continuing professional development (CPD) • The contribution of the portfolio to support student learning in practice • The portfolio as an assessment tool • Using the portfolio to assess competence • Conclusion • Summary of key points • Recommended further reading • References

Introduction

In outlining the purpose of portfolios, it is important first to examine the exact nature of a portfolio and its uses to date. In their paper on the subject (Rassin *et al.* 2006), a general background and definition is provided of 'portfolio', with an interesting derivation of the term. It is suggested that the word portfolio originates from the Italian word 'portare fogliou' which means to carry paper (Rassin *et al.* 2006). Portfolios have been used extensively in other professions such as artistry, photography, architecture and music for several decades (Serembus 2000; Lettus *et al.* 2001; Rassin *et al.* 2006). The interest in portfolios as a tool for educational purposes in nursing developed in the mid-1980s (Rassin *et al.* 2006). Many Schools of Nursing now use portfolios as a method of both formative and summative assessment (Rassin *et al.* 2006).

Within nursing practice portfolio use is also a widely accepted method of recording professional development for qualified nurses. This concurrent use within the profession, as both an educational tool and a means of recording ongoing professional development, while exemplary, can lead to confusion. This chapter clarifies and defines portfolio use within nurse education and considers its use both to assess and develop student learning in this context.

> Portfolios have been identified as a means to carry items. They are in widespread use in professions such photography, architecture and music.

Defining 'portfolio'

As you read in Chapter 1, in keeping with a shifting emphasis towards self-directed learning among nursing students, portfolios are widely accepted as a valuable learning tool within nurse education (Kelly 1996). Their use and development are also increasingly becoming a fundamental part of professional nursing career development (Rassin *et al.* 2006). The literature is replete with descriptions and definitions of portfolio (Brown 1992; Price 1994; Hull *et al.* 2005) and there is often ambiguity regarding differentiation between the terms profile and portfolio. According to Redman (1994: 11) 'a portfolio is simply a tangible record of what someone has done'. This would appear to suggest that a portfolio merely accounts for achievements to date, whereas a portfolio can be further defined as a collection of evidence attesting to knowledge and skill development (Brown 1992). The latter is the most commonly accepted definition (Jasper 2003) of a portfolio within the context of nursing, revealing the portfolio to be a 'private collection of evidence which demonstrates the continuing acquisition of skills, knowledge, attitudes, understandings and achievements. It is both retrospective and prospective, as well as reflecting the current stage of development and activity' (Brown 1992: 3).

This later definition is more consistent with the dynamic nature of a portfolio that some authors recommend (Hull and Redfern 1996). However, difficulties emerge when considering these accepted definitions of portfolio for use in education settings as they apply more aptly to portfolios that are developed by qualified nurses as a record of their continuing professional development (CPD). This is clearly evidenced throughout key texts on the topic that focus solely on qualified nurses (Hull and Redfern 1996). More specific definitions will be considered later.

First, in demystifying what a portfolio is or can be for you as a student, clarity is required with regard to profile definition. A profile is described as a selection of evidence that may be extracted from a portfolio to fulfil a specific need (Brown 1992). This may then be shown to others to fulfil a purpose, whereas the greater portion of the portfolio may remain private. Therefore, one could use a portfolio as a basis for a profile and develop an array of profiles to meet different, distinctive needs. The literature describing portfolio use among qualified nurses uses the terms 'personal portfolio', 'personal, professional portfolio' and 'professional portfolio' interchangeably (UKCC 1996; Hull *et al.* 2005; NCNM 2006; NMC 2006). For the purposes of this discussion the term portfolio will be used to describe a collection of evidence that attests to learning and knowledge among both nursing students and qualified nurses.

A portfolio is a collection of evidence that demonstrates learning and knowledge. A profile is a selection of this evidence that may be extracted to fulfil a particular purpose

---

With regard to the use of portfolio as a CPD tool, this facilitates qualified nurses to document their professional career outcomes, work experience and skills and may be used to market their skills positively in relation to job opportunities or promotion (Rassin *et al.* 2006). The portfolio as a mechanism for continuing professional development (CPD) will be briefly considered.

The portfolio as a mechanism for continuing professional development (CPD)

The use of a portfolio is described as an emerging method for practitioners to demonstrate and record competence (Storey 2001). Because the nurses' contributions are made over a period of time, the portfolio documents ongoing knowledge acquisition and skill proficiency, and the development of critical thinking and clinical decision making thus provide evidence of competency attainment. It is declared to be 'the quintessential evidence of commitment to continuing education and lifelong learning in nursing' (Billings and Kowalski 2005: 150). Furthermore, much of the literature asserts that the portfolio has the potential to transcend beyond professional development in that it links the development of the personal with the professional. Therefore portfolios can facilitate both personal and professional growth (McMullan *et al.* 2003).

In some countries, such as the United Kingdom (UK), keeping a portfolio or profile is a mandatory requirement of registration and portfolio use is increasingly becoming a fundamental aspect of the continuing professional development of nurses. Therefore as a nursing student in the UK, if you are fortunate enough to be using portfolios during your initial preparatory nurse education programme, this will be a useful introduction to portfolios, which will ultimately become an obligatory requirement of you as a registered nurse in later years. This has emerged since the 1990s, when registered nurses became obliged to undertake CPD and to provide evidence of this in their personal portfolio or profile in order to maintain their UK registration status (UKCC 1990; Hull and Redfern 1996). Post-registration education and practice (PREP) is maintained by the National Nursing and Midwifery Council, the regulatory body for nursing in the UK. PREP is a set of Nursing and Midwifery Council (NMC) standards and guidance which is designed to help provide the best possible care for patients and clients. In addition to 450 hours of practice, in order to re-register nurses and midwives must have undertaken at least five days (35 hours) of learning in the previous three years. This is the required standard of continued professional development (CPD) known as PREP (NMC 2006). Nurses and midwives are provided with broad guidelines for providing evidence that learning has taken place, and although they must declare their compliance to the requirements they are not required to show their profile or portfolio to the NMC or employers. Rather they may be selected to complete an audit form as part of the NMC's quality assurance initiative (NMC 2006).

Activity 1

List what you see as the benefits to the profession associated with registered nurses providing evidence of their learning and CPD.

List what you see as the benefits to individual nurses through their development of their portfolio.

You may write down your thoughts on this before proceeding with the chapter.

A similar situation operates within the United States of America (USA): in order to renew certification, evidence of both clinical practice and CPD are required (ANA 2007). A portfolio of achievement is not specifically required although it is suggested as a useful means of storing the relevant information (Wicker 2006). A template is provided for this, and it is suggested that this portfolio is brought to interviews and could include such things as 'Thank you' cards from patients (Wicker 2006). Furthermore, the centre for management of registration, the American Nurses Credentialing Center (ANCC), has a partnership with Decision Critical Inc. (DCI), a health care education company, to jointly market DCI's web-based professional portfolio management application – the Critical Portfolio™ (Anonymous 2006). This latter software, although not compulsory, may be purchased by nurses, and provides them with a framework for systematically outlining their CPD in order to assist them with renewing their practice certification. Decision Critical Inc. markets this Critical Portfolio™ (www.decisioncritical.com) and approximately 44,000 nursing students, who are members of the National Student Nurses Association, are using the application to plan their portfolios for their future nursing career (Anonymous 2006).

Activity 2

Log onto the Decision Critical Inc. www.decisioncritical.com website and select products, then critical portfolio.

Read through the information provided and consider the benefits of using a predesigned portfolio.

Although designed for registered nurses, do you see a structured electronic portfolio of this kind as something that may be useful to you as student?

Do you perceive any drawbacks with a structured electronic portfolio of this kind for nursing students?

Write down your observations.

Portfolios as evidence of CPD are used in a similar way by nurses and midwives in Australia, where there is an obligation to self-declare competence and fitness to practise when renewing annual practice certificates (Emden *et al.* 2003). Portfolio use is also suggested as a means of CPD for qualified nurses and students in Israel (Rassin *et al.* 2006). Although not linked to mandatory registration, a similar initiative has been implemented in the Republic of Ireland (NCNM 2003). This encouragement and support of portfolio development by qualified nurses occurs across the globe. This process is not necessarily linked to portfolios that are used within nurse education programmes, although the NMC recently suggested that nursing students upon completion of their education programme ought to have a portfolio that attests to their commitment to CPD (NMC 2004). Thus linkages and overlap between the processes are likely. For the moment, however, the portfolio as it is used to support student learning will now be considered exclusively.

The contribution of the portfolio to support student learning in practice

One of the incentives for portfolio introduction into nurse education, particularly in the UK, is to develop assessment strategies that will integrate theory with practice and thereby address the theory–practice divide (English National Board 1991; Crandall 1998; Gallagher 2001; Harris *et al.* 2001; McMullan *et al.* 2003). So in addition to a drive towards increased self-directed learning methods, there has long been concern among educators that gaps exist between classroom teaching and the clinical experiences that students have. Both modern nursing approaches and university systems provide a structure that entails long periods of study interspersed with clinical practice, so it can be a challenge for you as a student to think back on all your prior study and apply that to a clinical placement. The reflective component of the portfolio provides this link (Harris *et al.* 2001) through fostering skills of reflection, critical thinking and problem-solving by reflecting on clinical experiences in a structured, facilitated way. Linking portfolio assignments to clinical practice enhances programme credibility (Melrose 2006). A nursing student portfolio is a self-directed activity usually associated with clinical practice that is guided by facilitation. Following the diagnosis of learning needs, goals may be set and the student relevant activities outlined. The relevant activities depend on individual and course requirements and may include the provision of relevant competency assessment documentation and/or pieces of reflection. In addition to being a medium for recording learning achievements, a student portfolio can be a catalyst for growth by providing evidence not only of the product of your accomplishments, but also of the actual process of developing portfolios (Price 1994; Jasper 1995a; Crandall 1998; Wenzel *et al.* 1998). This can provide you with an in-depth knowledge both personally and professionally (Lettus *et al.* 2001). This can lead to awareness of your own skills, strengths and limitations as well as providing an indication of your developmental needs and a means for working on action plans to achieve future goals (Redman 1994; Priest and Roberts 1998; Wenzel *et al.* 1998; McMullan *et al.* 2003; Hull *et al.* 2005).

Activity 3

If you have experienced a period of intensive education within the Nursing School, think for a moment about the various topics that you have learned about and write them down (no need to refer to notes!). How many topics are you trying to remember in total?

Consider whether you perceive these as individualistic components of your education programme? Or are they consolidated within your thinking as one unit of learning (ie nursing)?

Think about your recent learning experiences in the clinical area. Does this lead you to reconsider these various topics?

Write down your observations.

It is generally agreed (Glen and Hight 1992; McMullan *et al.* 2003) that the theoretical basis for the portfolio includes the four assumptions of adult learners outlined by Knowles. These assumptions suggest the learner is self-directed, that past experiences are a rich resource for learning, that student readiness to learn develops from life tasks and problems and, finally, that the student demonstrates curiosity and is self-motivated to grow and achieve. While these concepts may seem essential to adult learning and are akin to portfolio development it must be acknowledged that not all students will ascribe to these concepts or demonstrate or display these tendencies. If the broader uses and potential of the portfolio in student nurse personal and professional development are to be envisaged then the potential to foster and enhance these tendencies can be nurtured through facilitation (Cayne 1997; Knowles *et al.* 1998).

The portfolio approach shifts the emphasis from that of passive teacher-led learning to a more student-led experiential type of education. The preceptor/ mentor or assigned registered nurse has an invaluable role to play in facilitating this process. This preceptor/mentor can help you to identify your own learning needs and goals by assessing your knowledge, level of competence development and ability to link practice with theory. Therefore the portfolio can be a method by which the link between theoretical learning and practical experience can be further facilitated through discussion (Harris *et al.* 2001) between you and the preceptor or mentor. By virtue of the nature of the portfolio being developed over a period of time, relationships can be developed which enable you to seek support and guidance at crucial times as your individual needs arise in order to maximize the portfolio as a learning tool for your personal and professional development. Learning can also be a reciprocal process in which the portfolio can provoke thought or incite learning opportunities in your facilitator too. This potential for learning to be enhanced through facilitation experiences is evident within the research literature (Ferguson 1996), with 'mentoring' experiences not only proving beneficial to students but having the potential to keep staff nurses more aware, focused and up to date (Atkins and Williams 1995). Karlowicz (2000) proposes that portfolio development encourages students and teachers to be partners in the educational process. The establishment of collaborative relationships is an important dimension to student portfolio. Critical analysis, for example, may be mastered by experienced practitioners or educationalists, but the development of critical thinking and ability to analyse critically and synthesize evidence may well be a developmental process within undergraduate students that needs to be fostered throughout their education pertinent to their level of training. As a novice learner and practitioner, the student nurse needs guidance and support in developing and using a portfolio, so it can be used as a medium for discussion of progress to date and future aspirations and goals in a sensitive, supportive, facilitative manner essential to the novice.

Activity 4

If you have worked with a preceptor/mentor or registered nurse during your clinical experiences, identify ways that this person helped to apply and understand your classroom learning.

Identify things that this mentor may have done that you believe enhanced your learning.

Write down your observations.

McMullan *et al.* (2003) suggest the portfolio attests to achievement and personal and professional development, by providing critical analysis of its contents. Similarly, it is suggested the portfolio at a minimum should illustrate a student's ability to think critically, perform appropriate therapeutic nursing interventions, and communicate effectively. Karlowicz (2000) also suggests that an overview of each document contained in the portfolio should be created by the student to describe and analyse specific accomplishments. Karlowicz proposes that this information will enhance, for example, the evaluators' understanding of the significance of a particular entry in the portfolio, as well as enable the student to rediscover the learning that has occurred and skills that have been acquired. This prevents the 'shopping trolley' approach that was mentioned in Chapter 1, in which contents haphazardly lie within the folder. If you write an overview of each document contained, this allows you to develop a train of thought that may permeate through your complete portfolio, or at least provides for some cohesion within. This also supports the notion of you as a student taking action and responsibility for portfolio contents and their relevance to your learning. Rather than each ward policy or teaching booklet or research article being explained to you by the nurse, you are responsible for reading, understanding, seeking out new information, putting it all together and making sense of your collected documents in context. This yields rich and valuable learning for the adult learner.

Practical problems associated with portfolio use in the clinical area include issues of appropriate and safe storage (Brooks *et al.* 1999) and the amount of time taken to complete (Snadden 1999; Harris *et al.* 2001). Unfortunately there is no quick fix to some of these highlighted concerns; if at all possible, it is best for you to try to locate a suitably safe place to store the portfolio on the clinical placement. This renders the portfolio easily accessible while on placement so that it can be used as near as possible to the time of clinical experiences, enabling you to make the most of your memory and the facilities available while on placement.

Students additionally express anxiety about the nature and amount of

Remember!

Take your portfolio with you at all times when on clinical placement and seek a suitable storage area to put it for safe keeping when you are not actively using it.

evidence to be provided (Mitchell 1994). This anxiety, together with the time-consuming aspect, may have a negative effect on students' motivation (Mitchell 1994). Students need guidance on how to use their portfolios (McMullan *et al.* 2003) and they may need suggestions at least initially regarding the types of evidence to include in the professional portfolio, which this book endeavours to achieve. Karlowicz (2000) proposes that a process be established that aids students in selecting documents or projects that effectively show the acquisition of competencies or behaviours. Students also need feedback regarding how they are progressing and suggestions to alleviate problems they may be experiencing. Many students find the notion of developing a portfolio daunting and overwhelming at first (Serembus 2000), especially the novice looking for a simple how-to guide. Establishing guidelines for students to follow can facilitate or ease this process.

> Portfolios can be perceived as a daunting and time-consuming task but are vehicles for rich and rewarding learning. Seek out simple guidelines about material for inclusion and remember to discuss/summarize or describe each artefact that you include.

Contemporary nurse education places emphasis on facilitating learning rather than didactic teaching and encourages greater student involvement and empowerment. It is argued that the student portfolio has the potential to be used as a way of facilitating students as autonomous learners and practitioners by encouraging them to take more responsibility for the direction, progress and quality of their learning as well as for the development of better study skills. It is postulated by Murrell *et al.* (1998) as a means of facilitating students in taking control of their own learning needs. This may generate anxiety in some students and may necessitate sensitive and supportive encouragement to foster essential qualities in the attainment of autonomy and accountability for professional practice. Some of this anxiety may relate to the extent to which a student is ready to be self directed. As discussed in Chapter 1, there are three elements to this readiness: self-management, desire for learning and self-control (Fisher *et al.* 2001). Lack of ability in any of these areas, but particularly self-management, could easily cause the portfolio to become an onerous task.

> ### Activity 5
>
> From our discussions about portfolios within the book so far, or from your own experiences, what are your views on their ability to generate greater student involvement and independence?
>
> Is this independence in learning a source of anxiety for you? Or a challenge?

If you were to complete a portfolio what steps would you take to lessen your own anxiety, if any?

Write out your observations.

A point that should remain at the forefront of the minds of all those involved in the formation of portfolios and its inherent expectations is highlighted by Jasper (1995b), who declares the integration of the whole experience should match the students' stage of professional and academic development. The concern, Jasper declares, is that overly complex approaches, particularly in the early stages of students' careers, can detract from clinical learning in favour of learning how to complete the portfolio successfully. The purpose of the portfolio is not to provide students with yet another daunting, anxiety-inducing task but rather to elicit interest in its use and development in students and foster an understanding and appreciation of its potential in their progress throughout their nursing education and beyond.

If, as Jasper suggests, you believe your portfolio expectation to be overly complex for your level of education, seek to address this locally through your student representation within the School.

It has been said many times that learning through the use and development of a portfolio is progressive where, for example, nursing students who begin a portfolio earlier in the nursing programme will be able to demonstrate learning over time (De Natale and Romeo 2000). While the benefits of portfolios are well documented within the discourse, so too are the difficulties. Therefore the progressive, iterative nature of the portfolio is arguably the essence of its value where learning and development takes place over a period of time at each individual's own pace and needs to be supported and guided according to each individual's needs.

Portfolio use within nursing practice in recent years has been extensive (Rassin *et al.* 2006). This includes use for both CPD and educational purposes (Rassin *et al.* 2006). Its use for the latter is promoted for both undergraduate and postgraduate levels. However, while there is a range of literature supporting and directing portfolio development for qualified nurses, as described above, there is a dearth of existent literature that addresses portfolios specifically from the nursing student's perspective (Brooks *et al.* 1999). It is primarily the remit of each educational establishment where portfolios are used to develop its own guidelines. Thus there is no consistent approach to their use. Available literature describes current portfolio structure in some areas and use for both undergraduate and postgraduate nursing students, ascertains students' views and discusses and debates the portfolio as both a learning and assessment tool for these groups, but offers little by way of direct guidance regarding the individual planning or management of student portfolios. In the UK, nursing students are required to develop a portfolio during their programme in order to satisfy the requirements for entry into the professional register (NMC 2004). Although specific guidelines regarding this portfolio construction are not provided it is suggested that it 'demonstrate a commitment to the need for continuing professional development' (NMC 2004: 5).

Core common components of portfolios include: a reflective student record of experiences including analysis and synthesis of learning from these situations including explanation of changes to opinions or behaviours as a result of reflection (Rassin *et al.* 2006). The portfolio may also include opinions of colleagues or grades (Rassin *et al.* 2006). Cooper (1999) identifies three distinct forms of portfolio within nurse education: the competency-based portfolio, the negotiated learning portfolio, and the biographic profile (Box 2.1). The *competency-based* portfolio is used in conjunction with the curriculum structure to provide for appropriate assessment of clinical performance. The *negotiated learning* portfolio involves negotiated learning outcomes. The outcomes of the negotiated learning processes are assessed using evidence submitted in a portfolio format. The *biographic* portfolio is a record of achievement. In this type of portfolio a student 'collects time-sequenced historically ordered evidence from a work experience placement about tasks that the student has undertaken' (Cooper 1999: 46). Of these typologies, the competency-based portfolio appears the most commonly described within the literature. The negotiated learning portfolio is rarely used (Cooper 1999), although this would fit nicely into the notion of self-directed learning. Similarly the biographic portfolio is rarely used.

Portfolios used in nurse education settings therefore have a wide range of purposes and functions and indeed vary greatly in their construction. Their uses include demonstration of knowledge, reflection purposes, as a component of formative and summative assessment, to develop critical thinking skills, to develop skills of writing and to integrate theory with practice (Jasper and Fulton 2005). In contrast to portfolios that are used for CPD, portfolios used within an educational context are required to have a significant theoretical component (Jasper and Fulton 2005). One main difference emerging from Brown's (1992) popular definition is with regard to the privacy of the portfolio. While this is true perhaps for qualified nurses, who may select a section

---

Box 2.1 Types of portfolio

- *Competency-based*
- *Negotiated learning*
- *Biographic*

Source: Cooper (1999).

or profile for particular uses, a portfolio that you may use as a student is usually submitted in its entirety and not privately kept, particularly when a component of assessment. From a literature review on the topic McMullan *et al.* (2003: 288) provide a fitting definition that may be used to guide further discussions: 'A portfolio is a collection of evidence, usually in written form, of both the products and processes of learning. It attests to achievement and personal and professional development, by providing critical analysis of its contents'.

Remember!

'A portfolio is a collection of evidence, usually in written form, of both the products and processes of learning. It attests to achievement and personal and professional development, by providing critical analysis of its contents' (McMullan *et al.* 2003).

There are several key words from within this definition that are crucial to the understanding and use of your student portfolio. Unlike qualified nurses, who may hold a range of certificates or have attended educational seminars, you as a nursing student await both your final transcript, outlining your achievements, and your award certificate from your educational establishment until your programme is complete. Therefore your collection of evidence as a student will vary considerably from that of the registered nurse. The evidence will first need to be relevant to the particular portfolio aims. Secondly, it needs to be valid evidence. It is not simply sufficient to place a published article, for example, into the portfolio as evidence.

Remember!

The evidence will first need to be relevant to the particular portfolio aims. Secondly, it needs to be valid evidence. It is not simply sufficient to place a published article, for example, into the portfolio as evidence.

The article (or other document) requires some discussion and/or critical analysis of its contents, as is suggested, to provide the relevant evidence (Karlowicz 2000). Evidence of achievement of competences may be relevant evidence in this context depending on the use of portfolios at your School. Another item that is often not fully developed within student portfolios is the cohesive approach (Karlowicz 2000). A cohesive approach concurs with Knowles's view that evaluation should form a component of any self-directed learning activity. This means that you would provide evaluative statements or summaries related to your reading and your learning. Similarly, a synthesis of learning within the portfolio is expected (Rassin *et al.* 2006), which suggests that you put ideas together. Thus your portfolio should knit together so that both evidence and critical analysis weave together to form the overall account (Jasper 2003). Within this section the relevant learning within the portfolio may be summarized and it may be ascertained whether or not your personal learning goals were achieved. As Lyons (1998: 5) suggests, 'the real power of a portfolio process . . . may well be in the acts of . . . constructing, presenting and reflecting on the . . . evidence'. Thus the interpretation and operation of your portfolio in practice moves from a mere collection to a cohesive construction and presentation that includes reflection on evidence. From these points, and the points raised in Chapter 1, McMullan *et al.*'s definition could be further expanded to suggest that:

> A portfolio is a collection and cohesive account of work-based learning that contains relevant evidence from practice and critical reflection on this evidence. Its primary purpose is to display the achievement of professional learning outcomes and knowledge development. However, an inherent aim is the encouragement of personal development.

Remember!

A portfolio is a collection and cohesive account of work-based learning that contains relevant evidence from practice and critical reflection on this evidence. Its primary purpose is to display the achievement of professional learning outcomes and knowledge development. However, an inherent aim is the encouragement of personal development.

Contemporary thought on portfolios declares that it has the potential to facilitate and achieve much more than mandatory guidelines might suggest. The literature is replete with its potential for growth, achievement, accomplishment and development containing evidence attesting to professionals' competence to practise their craft and explication of tacit knowledge (Serembus 2000). The portfolio is accredited with a wide variety of purposes (Billings and Kowalski 2005) (Table 2.1).

Contemporary portfolios can be viewed therefore as having many functions for both qualified and undergraduate nursing students preparing for professional practice. Being prescriptive about a portfolio, however, mitigates against its individual dynamic nature. Nonetheless, at undergraduate level it is necessary and important to be guided and supported in the development of a portfolio, rendering the process easier to follow by suggestions and guidelines for the organization, development and use of the portfolio.

Table 2.1 Purposes of portfolios

* Document learning.
* Demonstrate accomplishment of specified competencies or criteria.
* Identify strengths and areas for improvement.
* Showcase a career trajectory.
* Demonstrate how learning connects to practice outcomes.
* Plan transition into practice.
* Award financial merit.
* Empower nurses to take responsibility for their own learning.
* Provide a broader view of learning over time by linking experiences and skills to professional competency.
* Demonstrate knowledge that can be converted to academic credit.
* Serve as a starting point for planning and individualizing learning during orientation.
* Determine advanced placement or shortened orientation time and faster transition to the work force.
* Promote transition from academic to service setting by reviewing the new graduate's documented competencies and tailoring orientation programmes accordingly.

Source: Billings and Kowalski (2005).

Remember!

Contemporary portfolios can be viewed therefore as having many functions for both qualified and undergraduate nursing students preparing for professional practice.

This is illuminated through the use and development of a portfolio and the development and attainment of competence throughout the student nurses' undergraduate programme. Portfolios are accredited as a means to acknowledge the work achieved by students from diverse cultural and linguistic backgrounds as well as those with physical limitations (Lettus *et al.* 2001). The National Council for Nursing and Midwifery in the Republic of Ireland (NCNM 2003, 2006) suggest many uses of the portfolio, specifically that undergraduate nurses can use it to demonstrate learning and development of their skills of reflection and critical thinking. Nursing student portfolios are commonly used for assessment purposes and this aspect will now be further discussed.

Undergraduate nurses can use portfolios to demonstrate learning and development of their skills of reflection and critical thinking.

The portfolio as an assessment tool

Portfolio assessment is one of the tools being closely examined in the educational community as a method of authentic assessment. This form of assessment has the unique ability to capture learning over time in a way that excels that of standard examinations or traditional continuous assessment (Lettus *et al.* 2001). Portfolios may be used within education for both summative and formative purposes (Cooper 1997, 1999). Summative portfolios focus on learning outcomes and contain evidence that these were achieved. This measures students' skills or knowledge. Where the main role of a portfolio is to demonstrate the processes of learning the assessment is often formative (Cooper 1997, 1999).

Remember!

Portfolios that you are expected to complete as a component of a nursing programme may be awarded a mark/grade (summative) or not (formative).

However, there is debate within the literature about the effectiveness of portfolios as an assessment tool (Gerrish *et al.* 1997; Wenzel *et al.* 1998; Gannon *et al.* 2001; McMullan *et al.* 2003). Pearce (2003) suggests that the notion of portfolio and assessment is very broad and questions how they can best be used for this purpose. It is generally accepted that when linked to summative assessment this relates to providing evidence of achievement of curricular learning outcomes; there is also reference within the literature to assessment of competence by this means. Pearse suggests that there should be a greater focus within the assessment on the planning, collection and analysis within the portfolio (Pearce 2003).

There is general agreement on the value of portfolios for formative assessment, but little information on their use for summative assessment (Jasper 1995; Pitts *et al.* 1999; Snadden 1999; McMullan *et al.* 2003). Summative assessment of portfolios can adversely affect the extent to which you as a student experience ownership of this important tool, and as a result your full use of the portfolio may be discouraged. The portfolio may then become assessment-led, potentially resulting in a reduction in its learning value. Paradoxically, however, it is argued that you are less likely as a student to use or prepare your portfolio if it is not assessed (Harris *et al.* 2001; Dolan *et al.* 2004). In some Schools of Nursing formative assessment of portfolio occurs in the early years of the programme, with summative assessment taking the form of a portfolio-based essay rather than the submission and assessment of the portfolio *per se* (Pearce 2003).

In some Schools of Nursing formative assessment of portfolio occurs in the early years of the programme with summative assessment taking the form of a portfolio-based essay rather than the submission and assessment of the portfolio *per se*.

The problems associated with portfolio assessment are akin to some of those long-standing issues noted within clinical nursing practice assessment such as objectivity, validity, reliability, honesty and confidentiality (Karlowicz 2000; Gannon *et al.* 2001). Difficulty exists in proving that a score assigned to a student portfolio is measuring what it is intended to measure. Assessment can elicit reluctance in students to express their innermost thoughts and feelings, and the potential to view assessment as an invasion of their privacy exists. You as a student may be inclined to write what you think the assessor wants to read (Mitchell 1994; Gerrish *et al.* 1997; Snadden and Thomas 1998; Woodward 1998), which of course defeats the purpose of the portfolio as a learning and developmental tool and thus reduces its validity and credibility as an assessment tool (Gannon et al. 2001). Also, the uniqueness of a student's work does not easily lend itself to comparison across a student population.

Inter-rater reliability among the portfolio reviewers is another challenge. Consistency among the assessors, in light of the volume and uniqueness of work, can be difficult to achieve and maintain. Lettus (Lettus *et al.* 2001) suggests that a way to alleviate this difficulty might be the development of some standard portfolio requirements along with well-trained reviewers. Cooper (1999) proposes that assessment should be fitting (appropriate to its intended purpose); fair, thus minimizing unfair bias in assessment; efficient, thus efficient in terms of time and other costs; monitored, and designed in such a way as to include measures that permit its own evaluation and ensure that the assessment process functions as intended relative to the desired pedagogic outcomes. Quinn (2000) further suggests a marking criteria for portfolios using five key headings: presentation; clinical expertise; professional role; management/education and innovation. The portfolio should be:

- fitting;
- fair;
- efficient.

(Quinn 2000).

Marking criteria should include marks awarded under the following categories:

- presentation;
- clinical expertise;
- professional role;
- management/education;
- innovation.

(Quinn 2000).

These suggestions again would seem to militate against the uniqueness and individuality and freedom within your portfolio but would appear to address some of the highlighted issues, at least in the initial stages of portfolio development. Standard portfolio guidelines may prove useful with novice users if it is to be considered for assessment. Webb *et al.* (2003) address the issue of rigour in portfolio assessment. In particular they explore the issues of validity and reliability of portfolios as summative assessment tools, which they suggest are as yet unresolved. These concepts relate to the ability of markers to assess a product fairly that is so diverse and unique. Increasing validity and reliability of the process, particularly through the use of a marking grid, improves the fairness of the assessment process. Webb *et al.* put forward a framework (Table 2.2) to ensure rigour in the assessment process.

Increasing validity and reliability of the process, particularly through the use of a marking grid, improves the fairness of the assessment process.

Of particular interest in this table (2.2) is the referral to the tripartite arrangement, which is common in the UK. This involves completion of the final student assessment in the clinical area in the presence of both clinical staff and faculty/university staff. Clearly the supportive element is evident here. Positive outcomes from tripartite arrangements have been reported in the literature (Williams 2003; Joyce 2005). To increase satisfaction from portfolio use and ensure equity, a decision trail is also suggested that contains: explicit marking criteria, evidence from a variety of sources, quality assurance processes and external examination (Webb *et al.* 2003). There is some evidence in the literature of the development of these marking criteria at post-registration level (Cook *et al.* 2003; Jasper and Fulton 2005; Joyce 2005). One set of marking criterion examines portfolio achievement in a range of areas (Jasper and Fulton 2005) (Box 2.2). A grade is assigned according to the student's achievement in relation to critical understanding of the subject knowledge base; originality; ability to analyse complex situations; ability to act independently; the development of new insights; effective communication; insight and portfolio cohesiveness and presentation (Jasper and Fulton 2005). The overall grade is awarded where the majority of marks fall. Some areas may not be fully suited to undergraduates and may require adaptation for use. It is suggested that criteria can be developed both for use in marker assessment or student self-assessment. The awarding of a mark to a portfolio is recommended, and the recognition of the uniqueness of each portfolio is accepted and provided for within the criteria.

Alexander *et al.* (2002) outline a simple tool for evaluation of portfolios by both teaching (faculty) staff (Figure 2.1) and student self-evaluation (Figure 2.2). Student self-evaluation, as part of the assessment process, may be of

Table 2.2 Criteria for assessing portfolio evidence defined using criteria for evaluating qualitative research

Criterion	Definition	Portfolio evidence
Credibility	Data sources are identified and described accurately. Enhanced by: • Prolonged involvement • Persistent observation • Triangulation • Peer debriefing and member checks	Written evidence of experience and achievement • Extended placements • Day-to-day observation by assessor • Variety of evidence – reflective accounts, skills checklists, etc. • Tripartite meetings
Transferability	Generalisability of transfer of findings from a sample to the population or whole group	Double marking Moderation External examining Quality assurance processes – internal and external
Dependability	Linked to credibility – external checks possible via audit trail	Assessor verifies evidence Grading criteria are explicit and transparent in curriculum documentation and assessment handbooks Moderation External examining Quality assurance processes – internal and external
Confirmability	Data are linked to their sources so that users may check conclusions and interpretations	Written evidence by student Verification by assessor and at tripartite meetings
Adequacy and appropriateness of data	Enough data are collected to achieve saturation and demonstrate variability	Evidence collected continuously and in a variety of clinical settings
Verification with secondary informants	Confirmation or otherwise by informants	Verification by assessor Tripartite meetings Service user involvement
Multiple ruters	More than one person codes the data	Assessor involves clinical team in gathering evidence Academic checks portfolio
Audit trial	Comprehensive documentation of evidence to allow reconstruction of how conclusions were drawn	Portfolio pro formas Assessment guidelines

Source: Webb *et al.* (2003). (© Elsevier).

Box 2.2 Portfolio marking criteria

This portfolio demonstrates the achievement of the following:

	Unsat 40 %	satisfactory 50%	good 60%	excellent 70%
Originality in utilising knowledge base and methods of inquiry in practice				
The ability to assess complex situations and articulate problems				
Decision-making and professional judgement in planning strategies to deal with complex situations				
The ability to act autonomously in planning and implementation and use others appropriately				
The development of new insights which enhance and develop practice				
Independent, critical and reflective thinking				
Effective communication with professionals and non-professionals				
Personal insight and self-awareness, acknowledgement of own limitations				
Present the portfolio within a coherent structure, which contains all the required elements, including the use of English and referencing system				

Assess or to use an X.
Join the marks up to create a profile that will indicate areas of strength and weakness.

Source: Jasper and Fulton (2005).

interest to you as a student. The results were encouraging, helping students develop valuable portfolios and contributing towards preparation and interviewing for nursing positions after graduation.

In a study of the use of portfolios to assess competence, Scholes *et al.* (2004) report that lack of uniformity in the preparation of assessors could affect how individuals carry out assessments, and they warned of the significant time investment required by both student and assessor. So, in addition to clear and consistent guidelines, there is also a need for staff education and training in this regard, and where possible a consistency of markers. Lack of uniformity of preparation among staff may affect assessment

(Calman *et al.* 2002). Therefore, while the educational preparation for the role of assessor is important, this must be followed by opportunities to gain experience in carrying out assessments and the use of standardized assessment tools such as those outlined in the tables above to improve reliability of marking. There is also a need for ongoing support for assessors in carrying out their role (Flanagan *et al.* 2000), so that consistency in the assessment process is assured.

The portfolio could also be criticized for disadvantaging the academic if it is to be used as an assessment tool; potential assessors clearly need to consider the contents of the portfolio, their relevance and application to the practice placement and to the clientele rather than solely its academic precision. Consideration also needs to be afforded to the goal of the portfolio: is it another academic pursuit or a means through which development of competence can be demonstrated or illustrated? These factors can be incorporated into locally modified marking criteria. Either way, as professionals, student nurses do have an academic standard to achieve and maintain, whether this is acknowledged or awarded in the portfolio, or its assessment is what is being questioned. Interestingly, students' views on portfolio assessment are very positive (Tiwari and Tang 2003).

Portfolios can assist individual learning or be a means of larger scale assessment, or can fulfil both functions. Is it possible to assess portfolios if the work is not standardized? Does it need to be assessed or can the evidence or contents provided within the portfolio provide the means to demonstrate and illustrate the development and achievement of competence as part of an assessment process? The literature abounds with suggestions of overcoming some of the difficulties perceived or encountered through assessing portfolios.

Whether the portfolio should be assessed is still questionable and whether it should be formatively or summatively assessed or both is debatable. It is important to realize the importance of a formative portfolio. This is 'process-orientated' and allows you to grow both personally and professionally as well as documenting your journey, without having a formal examination or assessment, which occurs within the summative route (Price 1994; Kelly 1996). Similarly, the use of the portfolio is advocated by Karlowicz (2000) as an adjunctive method of assessment where consideration needs to be given to not only the end product but also the benefits and limitations of the process.

There is debate within the literature about whether a portfolio should be formatively or summatively assessed.

While consideration does need to be afforded to both the process and the product of the portfolio if it is being assessed, this would again appear to be a

FACULTY PORTFOLIO EVALUATION TOOL: BACCALAUREATE STUDENT

Directions: Place a number 1 to 5 (see scale below) in each blank to indicate response to student's portfolio. This should be an assessment based upon your review of the contents of the portfolio.

| Superior | Good | Satisfactory | Below Average | Not Evident |
| 5 | 4 | 3 | 2 | 1 |

.... 1. Current resumé suitable for use when seeking desired nursing position.

.... 2. Evidence of participation in pre-professional or professional organizations.

.... 3. Evidence of effective verbal communication skills.

.... 4. Evidence of effective written/computer communication skills.

.... 5. Evidence of performance as an effective team or group member.

.... 6. Evidence of therapeutic interventions through clinical performance, mission, service, or church involvement.

.... 7. Evidence of leadership in community, campus or professional activities.

.... 8. Evidence of satisfactory clinical skills.

.... 9. Evidence of critical thinking ability through projects, research, or writings.

.... 10. Evidence of satisfactory academic performance.

.... 11. Evidence of leadership activities in campus, clinical community, or professional organizations.

.... 12. Appropriate letters of reference or appreciation.

What aspect of the portfolio was most impressive?

What needs or deficits were identified?

Faculty Signature ....   Student Signature ....

Date ....   Date ....

Figure 2.1 Faculty survey portion of the evaluation

Source: Alexander *et al.* (2002) with permission of *Journal of Continuing Education in Nursing.*

STUDENT PORTFOLIO SELF-EVALUATION TOOL

Directions: Place a number 1 to 5 (see scale below) in each blank to indicate your response to the following. This should be based upon how you feel about yourself in these areas:

Superior 5	Good 4	Satisfactory 3	Below Average 2	Not Evident 1

.... 1. Do you feel that your current resumé is suitable for use when seeking desired nursing position?

.... 2. How would you rate your participation in pre-professional/professional organizations?

.... 3. How do you feel about your verbal communication skills?

.... 4. How do you feel about your written/computer communication skills?

.... 5. How do you feel about your ability to work in a group or team?

.... 6. How do you feel about your skill in therapeutic interventions as evidenced in clinical performance mission work, and service?

.... 7. How do you feel about your participation in community activities?

.... 8. How do you feel about your clinical experiences?

.... 9. How do you feel about your critical thinking skills as demonstrated in research, projects, journal writing, and clinical performance?

.... 10. How do you feel about your academic performance?

.... 11. How do you feel about your participation in leadership activities?

.... 12. How do you feel about your ability to obtain letters of reference or appreciation?

Which aspect of the portfolio do you feel is most impressive?

What needs can you identify?

Student Signature ....   Faculty Signature ....

Date ....   Date ....

Figure 2.2 The self-evaluation section for students

Source: Alexander *et al.* (2002) with permission of *Journal of Continuing Education in Nursing.*

subjective conclusion. The answer McMullan *et al.* (2003) propose might be to use formative assessment for the reflective part of the portfolio with the remainder of the portfolio being summatively assessed, taking into account the reliability and validity issues discussed previously. This would appear to address issues surrounding the use of reflection such as confidentiality and credibility, but thought must be afforded to who might facilitate this formative approach and whether it would be awarded a credit or not in an attempt to address the issues raised regarding honesty and credibility.

The evaluation of portfolios is uncharted territory that is being approached cautiously and requires further exploration and research to support and validate some of the suggestions for resolving the issues that surround its assessment within educational practices. The portfolio is often used as an adjunct to assess competence, or frequently as a reservoir within which to place such documentation. Its use in this context will be briefly discussed and elaborated in Chapter 4.

Using the portfolio to assess competence

While the assessment of student performance in the clinical area has long formed a major component of preparatory nurse education programmes, the particular notion of clinical 'competence' arose in North America and is not unique to the profession of nursing (Watson *et al.* 2002). The nursing literature abounds with discussions from the UK, USA and Australia concerning the complexity of competence and the broad spectrum of ways in which it can be defined, operationalized and assessed (Ashworth and Morrison 1991; Bradshaw 1997, 1998; Chambers 1998; Eraut 1998; Milligan 1998; Storey 2001). Much of the literature on competence reveals it to be a key agenda item in the UK, USA and Australia. The assessment of learning and competence lies at the heart of nursing education, with equal importance now being ascribed to both the theoretical and practical elements within nursing curricula.

The transition to approaches where the focus of assessment is to establish that of the development and attainment of competence in undergraduate nurses has influenced the introduction of a variety of assessment tools. One catalyst that has fuelled this transition to alternative methods of assessment can be attributed to the difficulties associated with traditional methods used to assess student nurses' performance and application of knowledge within the clinical setting, some of which have been previously addressed. Concerns persist regarding the subjectivity (Chapman 1999; Griffin 2001; Dolan 2003), risk of observer bias (Calman *et al.* 2002) and the validity and reliability of traditional methods of clinical assessment (Griffin 2001; Watson *et al.* 2002; McMullan *et al.* 2003). Competence-based approaches have been criticized as being paper-driven, bureaucratic (Storey 2001), and time-consuming (Wilson-Barnett *et al.* 1995), with problems noted in the language used in competency documentation (Neary 1999; Griffin 2001).

These findings are corroborated in a study by Calman *et al.* (2002), where students expressed the view that staff saw competence documentation as 'paperwork' and a 'tedious formality' rather than an integral part of their supervision and educational role. Little consensus has been achieved on a valid reliable assessment tool and the clinical assessment of students continues to pose challenges for nursing education. It is therefore not surprising that many educational institutions have experienced difficulties in developing effective assessment strategies.

Competency tools and documents for the development and assessment of competence within the clinical area have drawn from and are underpinned by a wide variety of theoretical frameworks such as Benner (2000), Steinaker and Bell (1979) and Bondy (1983) and have used domains of competence frameworks such as those advocated by national regulatory bodies (An Bord Altranais 2000; NMC 2004). Similarly, in describing a portfolio as a private collection of evidence, which demonstrates the continuing acquisition of skills, knowledge, attitudes, understanding and achievements, Brown (1992) incorporated the domains of learning that are deemed essential to competence and a necessary component when assessing one's development of competence. It can be envisaged how the portfolio can be a very useful means to demonstrate competence development and formulate part of the assessment of competence.

The portfolio has been advocated for use with approaches to competence. It is purported to be a dynamic tool that demonstrates competence, as it is being maintained and developed over time. The eclectic use of the portfolio, competence approaches and reflection have been accredited as having the ability to augment and facilitate students' development and their skills for competence development (Griffin 2001; Bell *et al.* 2002). Similarly, competence has been described as a continuum along which people can move backwards as well as forwards and it must be acknowledged that in any clinical situation competence can deteriorate if it is not maintained (Storey and Haigh 2002). The use of the portfolio seems a useful way, therefore, to demonstrate not only the development of competence but also its maintenance pertinent to the level the student has reached.

One of the most documented uses of the portfolio is the provision and storage of evidence to support learning that helps to illustrate competence development and as a possible means of assessing that competence. Students need guidance and suggestions with regard to the types of evidence to include in the portfolio (Serembus 2000; Dolan 2003) and concerning the importance of relevance and applicability of their choice of evidence to their learning needs and the client group they are currently caring for. Storey and Haigh (2002) emphasize how important it is that the centrality of the patient is not lost in the process of developing clinical competence.

Some theorists have argued for the effectiveness of reflection as a learning strategy for the development of clinical competence (Boud et al. 1985; Chambers 1998). As reflective practice is deemed to be an important facet in the development of clinical competence, one could assume that as part of the portfolio development, competence may be assessed at least partially by assessing reflective skills. It is suggested that the written journal is a valid assessment of the learner's reflective skills; however, caution is required here as this could be measuring the student's ability to think and to write which does not inherently imply competent clinical practice.

This notion is supported by Calman et al. (2002) who advocated caution when assuming that the quality of the students' written work in their portfolio could be viewed as a reflection of their performance in practice. This further affirms the need for somebody suitably placed in knowledge and experience to review the contents and evidence provided by students to ensure their ability to apply that evidence to their practice. The significance of the portfolio contents and evidence cannot be over-emphasized in contextualizing that evidence to the students' current learning environment.

One study reveals the portfolio to be an important focus for discussion to establish the students' acquisition and application of knowledge (Farrell 2004). In this study the portfolio is used in a variety of ways such as providing a focus for discussion about its contents and as a means of questioning students to establish their knowledge. It is also acknowledged by qualified nurse participants within this study that there is a need to talk through the contents of the portfolio with the student to establish its applicability to the practice placement and moreover to the patients within that placement. This may perhaps indicate that this applicability and relevance was not immediately apparent. However, the nurses still report value in this sharing and vocalizing of student learning in the context of facilitation.

An important facet of continuous assessment that could formulate an aspect of the formative process of competence assessment via the portfolio is that of learner self-assessment (Watson et al. 2002), in which learners are required to make judgements about their own performance (Chambers 1998), thus allowing them to identify their own strengths and weaknesses. This is an approach advocated by Alexander et al. (2002). The principles of learner self-assessment would appear to embrace some of the concepts akin to adult education and those of the portfolio that foster ownership of, and responsibility for one's own learning needs. Thus, self-assessment in nursing education could be a valuable means through which the evidence and contents of the portfolio could be assessed. This could provide a focus for open discussion regarding the portfolio as a developmental tool to enhance the student's competence development. Thus the use of learner self-assessment could be increasingly encouraged and evaluated in nurse educational settings.

Students need to be prepared to meet the demands of the future, as healthcare consumers are demanding proof of their providers' competence. A portfolio is a vehicle for demonstrating that competence to practise nursing. Although developing a portfolio can seem overwhelming, Serembus (2000) suggests that establishing guidelines for students to follow will ease the process. While critics might declare this as contravening the individual nature of the portfolio, it is necessary to provide some guidelines for novice users and this book endeavours to provide clear guidelines for students to use to render the preparation and use of portfolios easier.

Conclusion

Portfolios are increasingly being introduced both in postgraduate and undergraduate nursing education programmes as a fundamental part of a professional nursing education. Although maintaining a portfolio for qualified nurses is not a mandatory requirement in many countries, there is a move towards this requirement in some countries. Their use is increasingly advocated and included in undergraduate and postgraduate nurse educational programmes as a means to achieving professional competence and maintaining lifelong learning. This chapter provided a snapshot of the purpose of portfolios. It outlined the potential contribution of the portfolio to continuing professional development and compared this with its use within specific educational contexts. It examined the current use of the portfolio as an assessment tool within nurse education and approaches to the assessment of competence via portfolio were described. The potential contribution of the portfolio to supporting student learning in practice was provided that highlighted potential pitfalls and provided advice on the prevention of these.

Summary of key points

- A portfolio is a collection and cohesive account of work-based learning that contains relevant evidence from practice and critical reflection on this evidence.
- Its primary purpose is to display achievement of professional competence or professional learning outcomes and knowledge development. However, an inherent aim is the encouragement of personal development.
- It is important as a student to remember the 'cohesive account' required and attempt to draw your work together within the portfolio.
- There is debate within the literature about whether a portfolio should be formatively or summatively assessed.
- Marking criteria are useful when assessing a portfolio.

Recommended further reading

Hull, C., Redfern, L. and Shuttleworth, A. (2005) *Profiles and Portfolios: A Guide for Health and Social Care*, 2nd edn. Basingstoke: Palgrave Macmillan.

Jasper, M. (2006) *Professional Development, Reflection and Decision-Making*. Oxford: Blackwell Publishing.

References

Alexander, J. G., Craft, S. W. *et al.* (2002) The nursing portfolio: a reflection of a professional, *Journal of Continuing Education in Nursing*, 33(2): 55–9.

ANA (2007) American Nurses Association website http://www.nursingworld.org. Retrieved 25 April, 2007.

An Bord Altranais (2000) *The Code of Professional Conduct for Each Nurse and Midwife*. Dublin: An Bord Altranais.

Anonymous (2006) The American Nurses Credentialing Center and Decision Critical Inc. announce strategic business relationship, *NevadaRNformation*, May/June/July: 23.

Ashworth, P. and Morrison, P. (1991) Problems of competence-based nurse education, *Nurse Education Today*, 11(4): 256–60.

Atkins, S. and Williams, A. (1995) 'Registered nurses' experiences of mentoring undergraduate nursing students, *Journal of Advanced Nursing*, 21(5): 1006–15.

Bell, M. L., Heye, M. L. *et al.* (2002) Evaluation of a process-focused learning strategy to promote critical thinking, *Journal of Nursing Education*, 41: 175–7.

Benner, P. D. (2000) *From Novice to Expert: Excellence and Power in Clinical Nursing Practice*, Commemorative Edition. New Jersey: Prentice Hall.

Billings, D. and Kowalski, K. (2005) Learning portfolios, *The Journal of Continuing Education in Nursing*, 36(4): 149–51.

Bondy, K. N. (1983) Criterion-referenced definitions for rating scales in clinical evaluation, *Journal of Nursing Education* 22(9): 376–82.

Boud, D., Keogh, R. *et al.* (1985) Promoting reflection in learning: a model, in D. Boud, D. Walker and R. Keogh (eds) *Reflection: Turning Experience into Learning*. London: Kogan Page.

Bradshaw, A. (1997) Defining 'competency' in nursing (Part I): a policy review, *Journal of Clinical Nursing*, 6(5): 347–54.

Bradshaw, A. (1998) Defining 'competency' in nursing (Part II): an analytical review, *Journal of Clinical Nursing*, 7(2): 103–11.

Brooks, B. A., Madda, M. *et al.* (1999) How to organize a professional portfolio for staff and career development, *Journal for Nurses in Staff Development (JNSD)*, 15(1): 5–10.

Brown, R. A. (1992) *Portfolio Development and Profiling for Nurses*. Lancaster: Quay Publishing.

Calman, L., Watson, R. *et al.* (2002) Assessing practice of student nurses: methods, preparation of assessors and student views, *Journal of Advanced Nursing*, 38(5): 516–23.

Cayne, J. V. (1997) Portfolios: a developmental influence?, in P. Abbott and R. Sapsford (eds) *Research into Practice: A Reader*. Buckingham: Open University Press.

Chambers, M. A. (1998) Some issues in the assessment of clinical practice: a review of the literature, *Journal of Clinical Nursing*, 7(3): 201–8.

Chapman, H. (1999) Some important limitations of competency-based education with respect to nurse education: an Australian perspective, *Nurse Education Today*, 19(2): 129–35.

Cook, S. S., Kase, R. *et al.* (2003) Portfolio evaluation for professional competence: credentialing in genetics for nurses, *Journal of Professional Nursing*, 19(2): 85–90.

Cooper, T. (1997) *Portfolio Assessment: A Guide for Students*. Perth: Praxis Education.

Cooper, T. (1999) *Portfolio Assessment: A Guide for Lecturers, Teachers and Course Designers*. Perth: Praxis Education.

Crandall, S. E. (1998) Portfolios link education with practice, *Radiologic Technology* 69(5): 479–82.

De Natale, M. L. and Romeo, R. H. (2000) Portfolios: documenting learning in a personal way, *Nurse Educator*, 25(2): 69–75.

Dolan, G. (2003) Assessing student nurse clinical competency: will we ever get it right?, *Journal of Clinical Nursing* 12(1): 132–41.

Dolan, G., Fairbairn, G. *et al.* (2004) Is our student portfolio valued?, *Nurse Education Today*, 24(1): 4–13.

Emden, C., Hutt, D. *et al.* (2003) Exemplar. Portfolio learning/assessment in nursing and midwifery: an innovation in progress, *Contemporary Nurse*, 16(1–2): 124–32.

English National Board (1991) *Professional Portfolio*. London: English National Board.

Eraut, M. (1998) Concepts of competence, *Journal of Interprofessional Care*, 12(2): 127–39.

Farrell, M. (2004) Illuminating the essential elements of the competence-based approach to nurse education through an exploration of staff nurses' experiences of its implementation within the practice placement: a phenomenological study. Unpublished Masters thesis, School of Nursing and Midwifery, University College Dublin.

Ferguson, L. M. (1996) Preceptors' needs for faculty support, *Journal of Nursing Staff Development*, 12(2): 73–80.

Fisher, M., King, J. *et al.* (2001) Development of a self-directed learning readiness scale for nursing education, *Nurse Education Today*, 21(7): 516–25.

Flanagan, J., Baldwin, S. and Clarke, D. (2000) Work-based learning as a means of developing and assessing nursing competence, *Journal of Clinical Nursing*, 9(3): 360–68.

Gallagher, P. (2001) An evaluation of a standards based portfolio [corrected and republished article originally printed in *Nurse Education Today*, 21(3), April 2001: 197–200].

Gannon, F. T., Draper, P. R. *et al.* (2001) Putting portfolios in their place, *Nurse Education Today*, 21(7): 534–40.

Gerrish, K., McManus, M. *et al.* (1997) *Levels of Achievement: A Review of the Assessment of Practice*. London: English National Board for Nursing, Midwifery and Health Visiting.

Glen, S. and Hight, N. F. (1992) Portfolios: an 'effective' assessment strategy?, *Nurse Education Today*, 12(6): 416–23.

Griffin, C. (2001) *The Development of Competencies for Registration*. Assessment of Competence Conference. Dublin: An Bord Altranais.

Harris, S., Dolan, G. *et al.* (2001) Reflecting on the use of student portfolios, *Nurse Education Today*, 21(4): 278–86.

Hull, C., Redfern, J. *et al.* (2005) *Profiles and Portfolios: A Guide for Health and Social Care*. Basingstoke: Palgrave Macmillan.

Hull, C. and Redfern, L. (1996) *Profiles and Portfolios: A Guide for Nurses and Midwives*. Basingstoke: Macmillan.

Jasper, M. (1995a) The portfolio workbook as a strategy for student-centred learning, *Nurse Education Today*, 15(6): 446–51.

Jasper, M. (1995b) The use of a portfolio in assessing professional education, in G. Gibbs (ed.) *Improving Student Learning: Through Assessment and Evaluation*. Oxford: Oxford Centre for Staff Development.

Jasper, M. (2003) *Beginning Reflective Practice: Foundations in Nursing and Health Care*, Cheltenham: Nelson Thornes.

Jasper, M. A. and Fulton J. (2005) Marking criteria for assessing practice-based portfolios at masters' level, *Nurse Education Today*, 25(5): 377–89.

Joyce, P. (2005) A framework for portfolio development in postgraduate nursing practice, *Journal of Clinical Nursing*, 14(4): 456–63.

Karlowicz, K. A. (2000) The value of student portfolios to evaluate undergraduate nursing programs, *Nurse Educator*, 25(2): 82–7.

Kelly, J. (1996) The really useful guide to portfolios and profiles, *Nursing Standard*, 10: 36.

Knowles, M., Holton, E. *et al.* (1998) *The Adult Learner: The Definitive Classic in Adult Education and Human Resource Development*, 5th edn. Houston, TX: Gulf Publishing.

Lettus, M. K., Moessner, P. H. *et al.* (2001) The clinical portfolio as an assessment tool, *Nursing Administration Quarterly*, 25(2): 74–9.

Lyons, N. (1998) *With Portfolio in Hand: Validating the New Teacher Professionalism*, New York: Teachers College Press.

McMullan, M., Endacott, R. *et al.* (2003) Portfolios and assessment of competence: a review of the literature, *Journal of Advanced Nursing*, 41(3): 283–94.

Melrose, S. (2006) Creating a psychiatric mental health portfolio: an assignment activity that works, *Nurse Education in Practice*, 6(5): 288–94.

Milligan, F. (1998) Defining and assessing competence: the distraction of outcomes and the importance of educational process, *Nurse Education Today*, 18(4): 273–80.

Mitchell, M. (1994) The views of students and teachers on the use of portfolios as a learning and assessment tool in midwifery education, *Nurse Education Today*, 14(1): 38–43.

Murrell, K., Harris, L. *et al.* (1998) Using a portfolio to assess clinical practice, *Professional Nurse*, 13: 220–3.

NCNM (2003) *Guidelines for Portfolio Development*. Dublin: National Council for the Professional Development of Nursing and Midwifery.

NCNM (2006) *Guidelines for Portfolio Development for Nurses and Midwives*. Dublin: National Council for Nursing and Midwifery.

Neary, M. (1999) Preparing assessors for continuous assessment, *Nursing Standard*, 13(18): 41–7.

NMC (2004) *Standards of Proficiency for Pre-registration Nursing Education*. London: Nursing and Midwifery Council.

NMC (2006) *The PREP Handbook*. London: NMC.

Pearce, R. (2003) *Profiles and Portfolios of Evidence*. Cheltenham: Nelson Thornes.

Pitts, J., Coles, C. *et al.* (1999) Educational portfolios in the assessment of general practice trainers: reliability of assessors, *Medical Education*, 33(7): 515–20.

Price, A. (1994) Midwifery portfolios: making reflective records, *Modern Midwife*, 4: 35–8.

Priest, H. and Roberts P. (1998) Assessing students' clinical performance, *Nursing Standard*, 12(48): 37–41.

Quinn, F. M. (2000) *The Principles and Practice of Nurse Education*, 4th edn. Cheltenham: Nelson Thornes.

Rassin, M., Silner, D. *et al.* (2006) Departmental portfolio in nursing – an advanced instrument, *Nurse Education in Practice*, 6(1): 55–60.

Redman, W. (1994) *Portfolios for Development: A Guide for Trainers and Managers*. London: Kogan Page.

Scholes, J., Webb, C. *et al.* (2004) Making portfolios work in practice, *Journal of Advanced Nursing*, 46(6): 595–603.

Serembus, J. F. (2000) Teaching the process of developing a professional portfolio, *Nurse Educator*, 25(6): 282–7.

Snadden, D. (1999) Portfolios – attempting to measure the unmeasurable?, *Medical Education*, 33(7): 478–9.

Snadden, D. and M. L. Thomas (1998) Portfolio learning in general practice vocational training – does it work?, *Medical Education*, 32(4): 401–6.

Steinaker, N. and M. R. Bell (1979) *The Experiential Taxonomy: A New Approach to Teaching and Learning*. London: Academic Press.

Storey, L. (2001) *The Concept of Competence*. Proceedings of the Assessment of Competence, Dublin: An Bord Altranais.

Storey, L. and Haigh, C. (2002) Portfolios in professional practice, *Nurse Education in Practice*, 2(1): 44–8.

Tiwari, A. and Tang, C. (2003) From process to outcome: the effect of portfolio assessment on student learning, *Nurse Education Today*, 23(4): 269–77.

UKCC (1990) *The Post Registration Education and Practice Project (PREP)* London: United Kingdom Central Council.

UKCC (1996) PREP and profiling. *Register*, 17: 7–10.

Watson, R., Stimpson, A. *et al.* (2002) Clinical competence assessment in nursing: a systematic review of the literature, *Journal of Advanced Nursing*, 39(5): 421–31.

Webb, C. R., Endacott, R. *et al.* (2003) Evaluating portfolio assessment systems: what are the appropriate criteria?, *Nurse Education Today*, 23(8): 600–9.

Wenzel, L. S., Briggs, K. L. *et al.* (1998) Portfolio: authentic assessment in the age of the curriculum revolution, *Journal of Nursing Education*, 37(5): 209–12.

Wicker, T. (2006) Do you need a professional portfolio?, *Arizona Nurse*, 59(5): 12.

Williams, M. (2003) Assessment of portfolios in professional education, *Nursing Standard* 18(8): 33–7.

Wilson-Barnett, J., Butterworth, T. *et al.* (1995) Clinical support and the Project 2000 nursing student: factors influencing this process, *Journal of Advanced Nursing (Print)*, 21(6): 1152–8.

Woodward, H. (1998) Reflective journals and portfolios: learning through assessment, *Assessment and Evaluation in Higher Education*, 23(4): 415–23.

3

Reflection and Reflective Writing

Fiona Timmins

Introduction • Background to reflection in nursing • Models of reflection • Reflective writing • Ethical and legal issues • Conclusion • Summary of key points • Recommended further reading • References

Introduction

From Chapter 2 we discover that a portfolio is a collection and cohesive account of work-based learning that contains relevant evidence from practice and critical reflection on this evidence. Pearce (2003: 20), in discussion of the portfolio, recognizes reflection as an 'effective tool for recognizing formal and informal learning and development through practice'. The portfolio should develop as a collection of evidence of both the products and processes of learning (McMullan *et al.* 2003). In addition, Lyons (1998) draws attention to reflection on evidence within the portfolio as an essential element. Reflection forms a key component of much of today's contemporary portfolio development (McMullan *et al.* 2003) and for this reason it is worth considering the origins of reflection within nursing and the potential contribution of models of reflection currently in use.

> - The portfolio should develop as a collection of evidence of both the products and processes of learning.
> - Reflection on evidence within the portfolio is an essential element.

Reflection and reflective practice emerged in the nursing literature in the late 1980s and early 1990s. Much of this work is based on the seminal writings of Dewey (1933) and Schön (1983). The terms have become embedded in professional nursing literature and guidelines; for example, the English National Board for Nurses (1994) advocate that student nurses should use reflection to learn from experience (Jarvis 1992). For registered nurses, the National Health Service Management Executive (1993) and United Kingdom Central Council for Nursing Midwifery and Health Visiting (UKCC 1996) advocate the use of reflection to support professional practice.

> Reflection and reflective practice emerged in the nursing literature in the late 1980s and early 1990s. Much of this work is based on the seminal writings of Dewey (1933) and Schön (1983).

Reflection is a process of deep thought that includes looking backwards to the situation being pondered upon and projecting forward to the future. It involves the skills of both recall and reasoning (Jarvis 1992). However, while reflection is a natural human thinking process, the deliberate and systematic use of reflection as a learning tool in professional practice is a complex activity (Burns and Bulman 2000). Several definitions of reflection emerge, with no consensus of opinion. Within professional education, Boud *et al.* (1985) suggest that reflection has a specific meaning 'relating to a complex and deliberate process of thinking about and interpreting experience in order to learn from it'. The National Health Service Management Executive (1993) describes reflection as a 'process' that describes, analyses and evaluates an experience. Moon (1999) suggests reflection is a set of abilities and skills for problem-solving while Kim (1999) has indicated that 'reflection is a process of consciously examining what has happened in terms of thoughts, feelings and actions against underlying beliefs, assumptions and knowledge as well as against the backdrop (i.e. the context or the stage) in which specific practice has occurred'. The lack of a clear definition of reflection, together with the plethora of terms used interchangeably in the literature, make this phenomenon difficult to utilize (Teekman 2000; Carroll *et al.* 2002).

Activity 1

Define reflection as you understand it

> Can you consider any benefits to your own personal reflection?
>
> Can you consider any drawbacks to your own personal reflection?
>
> Write down your observations before proceeding with the chapter.

One further criticism levelled at reflection is the dearth of empirical evidence supporting its usefulness in practice (Carroll *et al.* 2002), although Rolfe later put up a strong case in its defence (Rolfe 2005). Some would suggest that the notion of reflection and reflective practice has gained credence in the nursing profession due to its eagerness to build a body of knowledge specific to nursing (Carroll *et al.* 2002). However, reflection as a concept has more far-reaching origins.

> Nursing student reflection is encouraged to support developing skills of professional practice.

Background to reflection in nursing

Since the advent of critical social theory humans have been encouraged to reflect critically upon their experiences in a social context as a means of knowledge procurement. Critical theory emerged from a prominent Frankfurt School of thought, in the early part of the last century, led by German social scientists such as Theodor Adorno and Max Horkheimer, and most notably Jürgen Habermas (Calhoun 1995). While positivistic science sought factual information, critical theory began to explore people's experiences of those facts, particularly in a social context (Calhoun 1995). Critical theory espouses a critical engagement with the person's social world; a critical account of both historical and cultural conditions and a continuous re-examination of one's own understanding (Calhoun 1995). Habermas (1971) was particularly concerned with the dominance of positivism, and encouraged systematic reflection and self-understanding as an alternative form of knowledge development (Held 1980).

> ### Activity 2
>
> Positivism is concerned with scientific facts whereas critical theory relies on people's personal interpretations of facts and occurrences. The sun going down each night has a scientific explanation.

Consider your own personal interpretation of the next sunset that you experience. Write down your thoughts.

Consider the type of information that you would have if you added your story to several other stories of your family and friends. What type of information would this glean? Ask your friends to write their experience of a sunset and share this with one another.

Habermas (1971) argues that rather than the existence of one type of knowledge (positivism), there were three broad distinctions of knowledge. Empirical, guided by an interest in manipulation and control (positivism); interpretive, guided by a practical interest in subjective understanding rather than control; and emancipatory, guided by a reflexive interest that allowed humans to have greater autonomy (How 2003). Critical theory is concerned with understanding and applying meaning to the world and events, particularly in the social context in which they take place.

While positivistic science sought factual information, critical theory began to explore people's experiences of those facts, particularly in a social context (Calhoun 1995). Critical theory is concerned with understanding and applying meaning to the world and events, particularly in the social context in which they take place.

Critical theory supports the notion that personal reflection on events, in their social context, is a valid form of knowledge development. Rather than direct application of critical theory, it is the legacy of critical theory and its contribution to reflection that are influential in the development of portfolios within nurse education (Moon 1999). In relation to portfolio use, four fundamental components of critical theory can be useful to consider: the validity of interpretive and reflexive knowledge; the search for meaning and understanding as a legitimate form of enquiry; the importance of context and the centrality of reflection to the process of knowledge development. As the student portfolio aims to provide a collection of evidence that attests to student personal learning (McMullan *et al.* 2003), interpretive and reflexive learning gain importance. Similarly, the legacy of critical theory requires a search for meaning and this is central to the portfolio journey as the student struggles to make sense and put together learning from nursing practice. Reflection is central and it forms a major component of many portfolios. Ultimately, although not always explicitly stated, the portfolio is primarily aimed at knowledge development for the user.

Activity 3

Within the portfolio process the validity of interpretive and reflexive knowledge; the search for meaning and understanding as a legitimate form of
enquiry; the importance of context and the centrality of reflection to the process
of knowledge development are considered important.

Think back to Activity 2. The validity of interpretive knowledge is supported
here, as you and your family's experiences of sunset become important, in
addition to the scientific principles. Life is not merely a set of scientific principles; people's enjoyment of a sunset can add meaning to life and this is
important. Context is also important. A person just released from prison for
example would experience a sunset in a completely different way from those
for whom it is commonplace.

In addition to the concept of self-direction as discussed in Chapter 1, reflection
plays a central part of portfolio development. Many nursing student portfolios
encourage students to reflect on their practice. *Reflection* therefore contributes
to the conceptual framework for the developing portfolio. Many authors
espouse reflection as a key component of portfolio development (Moon 1999;
McMullan *et al.* 2003). A large variety of approaches to reflection are used
within a portfolio.

Activity 4

If you are using or familiar with using a model of reflection within your Nursing
School, identify the model_____

What are the component parts of this model?

What are the origins of this model?

Do you find it useful?

Is this/would this be useful for use within a portfolio?

Consider your answer before moving on in the chapter.

You have listed above the model of reflection that you are most familiar with.
Schools have various rationales for selecting models for use, but rather than an
ad hoc approach, as rigorous a system as possible needs to be employed in
selecting the best approach to use for reflection within the portfolio. The literature abounds with references to the difficulty with portfolio assessment due
to issues of reliability and validity, so considering the most robust system for
use seems appropriate. Indeed, Rolfe *et al.* (2001) suggest the use of *appropriate*
frameworks with the development of suitable estimations of rigour. Just as
there are differences in opinion regarding definitions of reflection, there are

divergent views regarding model use. Indeed, there is sparse direction regarding how to select an appropriate model. The selection ultimately requires a critical analysis of models of reflection.

> Just as there are differences in opinion regarding definitions of reflection, there are divergent views regarding model use. Indeed, there is sparse direction regarding how to select an appropriate model of reflection.

Models of reflection

When considering conceptual models of nursing for use in practice, Fawcett (1995) suggests first analysing and evaluating several existing models. This process could equally be applied to a selection of a model of reflection. She further suggests comparing the content of each conceptual model with a mission statement or philosophy, selecting the closest match. In applying this approach to portfolio use, models of reflection may be critically analysed to assess the extent of their fittingness to the aims of a portfolio. The ultimate aim of a student's portfolio is learning and knowledge development. Reflection is a complex and deliberate process that may be applied within the portfolio to these products and processes in order to interpret the meaning and to extract relevant learning (Boud *et al.* 1985: 10). The aim of this chapter is to consider the usefulness of currently used models of reflection in relation to the extent to which they may fulfil the portfolio aim. It is not within the scope of this book to describe all existing models, as most models of reflection are comprehensively described in other texts. The suggested reading list provides further guidance in this regard. While some suggestions are provided in this chapter and in Chapter 5 regarding model selections, this may remain a personal student choice or one within the educational establishment, according to educational aims or preferences.

To support an estimate of rigour and appropriateness of a model of reflection, Fawcett's categories for analysing the usefulness of conceptual models to guide nursing practice are used. These categories suggest close attention to the following: explication of origins, comprehensiveness of content, logical congruence, generation of theory, and credibility. The two initial categories, explication of origins and comprehensiveness of content, will be discussed here in line with a broad discussion of reflection. Logical congruence, generation of theory and credibility will be further discussed in Chapter 5 when considering the selection of a framework for reflection. Use of these categories provides a comprehensive framework for analysis of selected models (Fawcett 1995). To provide data for the analysis, a literature search was undertaken utilizing the article title index of the CINAHL database. Key terms used were reflection, [or] critical reflection, [or] models of reflection. The search spanned the complete database period (1982–2006). This yielded 563 citations. From an exploration of the complete reference lists, several seminal references and commonly used models of reflection emerged. These latter subsequently informed a critical analysis of models of reflection, using Fawcett's categories. Findings within each of these categories will be discussed sequentially.

Explication of origins

Fawcett suggests that explanation and understanding of the origins of the conceptual model ought to guide selection. Within nursing the origins of reflection have their roots in the seminal work of Dewey (1933), Kolb (1984) and Schön (1983). From a historical perspective Dewey (1933) first began to articulate the need to think reflectively in order to solve problems (Rolfe *et al.* 2001; Høyrup and Elkjaer 2006). However, it was not until the 1980s that reflection began to emerge as a popular mechanism for professional development (Mackintosh 1998; Høyrup and Elkjaer 2006). Schön, in particular, concerned with professionals' development of skills and knowledge, outlines reflection *in* and *on* action. Schön's conceptualization of reflection has been influential within the nursing profession, suggesting less reliance on traditional and scientific forms of enquiry and encouraging practitioners to learn from reflecting both within practice and on their practice (Rolfe *et al.* 2001). Opposed to the dominance of positivism, Schön proposes reflection as an alternative method of practice theory generation. Schön's seminal work subsequently underpinned many structured models of reflection for nursing practice (Rolfe *et al.* 2001). Schön's influence on reflection use is supported in the literature search: 20 per cent of papers referred to his seminal text in their discussions. Only 6 per cent made references to Dewey while 4 per cent referred specifically to Kolb.

Origins of reflection

- Dewey (1933)
- Kolb (1984)
- Schön (1983)

Reflection is also widely utilized as a teaching and learning methodology for nursing students. Kolb (1984) describes a model for experiential learning within the classroom that is widely used in nurse education (Brackenreg 2004). In the portfolio process, Kolb's learning cycle is popular as a framework to promote learning, as it brings together theory (reflection/conceptualization) and practice (experience/testing out) (McMullan *et al.* 2003). However, Kolb's cycle of learning has been criticized by those who argue that the use of this experiential cycle is again dependent on the individual factors such as the learner's interest and willingness to learn (Hull and Redfern 1996). Drawing upon the work of Kolb, Gibbs (1988: 46) further describes experiential learning methods for the classroom followed by a 'structured debriefing' exercise, commonly referred to as a model of reflection. The later model became popular for use within nurse education settings (Rolfe *et al.* 2001) and is widely used for educational purposes (O'Donovan 2006). Gibbs's model is cited by 4 per cent of papers in the literature and is primarily an educational framework (Rolfe *et al.* 2001) for use in teaching environments. Its use is suggested for reflection within nurse profile development (Hull *et al.* 2005).

Some models of reflection such as Gibbs (1988) were designed specifically with educational purposes in mind.

From the above analysis particular trends of origins begin to emerge that influence appropriate selection for use within a portfolio. First, reflection has been predominantly incorporated within nursing as a mechanism for the development of the individual professional in his or her own practice, largely influenced by Schön's (1983) notion of reflection *in* and *on* action. Models such as Kim (1999) and Taylor (2000, 2006), though influenced extensively by critical theory, retain this notion of individual professional self-development (Rolfe *et al.* 2001). Similarly aimed at self-development is Johns's (1999, 2004) model, influenced by Schön (1983) but drawing comprehensively upon Carper's (1978) ways of knowing. Kim Taylor and Johns are popular models chosen by practitioners for reflection upon practice, cited in 3 per cent, 7 per cent and 15 per cent of papers in the literature search respectively. However, although not specifically referring to particular authors (other than Schön 1983), contemporary authors raise concern with the individualized perspective that these models utilize (Boud *et al.* 2006), suggesting instead a greater focus on the context within which learning takes place. A criticism of these individual focused models of reflection is that they lack this critical perspective (Barnett 1997). Their orientation is overtly personal, often resulting in personal introspection rather than seeking to modify understandings in the domain of practice or indeed challenge the particular context and instigate wider change. While context may be referred to within particular models such as Taylor (2000, 2006), the focus is predominately self-development rather than taking action within a particular context.

Reflection has been predominantly incorporated within nursing as a mechanism for the development of the individual professional in his or her own practice largely influenced by Schön's (1983) notion of reflection in and on action.

The individual approach to reflection, which is ultimately about personal growth and development, is limited in its social contextual consideration and also lacks an overt action perspective (Barnett 1997). The extent to which such a personalized approach can relate to the measurement of competence in nursing practice is, therefore, questionable. Approaches to competence assessment generally prescribe domains or standards of practice, expected from the student, that indicate the optimal behaviours, attributes and actions as they occur in the world of practice. That is, they may be experienced and observed in the world of practice. Consequently reflection itself ought to be grounded in practice rather than the individual. One further difficulty with the individualistic approach to reflection used by nursing students is the potential narcissistic effect. The student is encouraged to describe a situation or event purely from his or her own perspective with little or no consideration of the wider context within which it took place:

> this is where problems occur. On the one hand, portfolios enable the student-writer to construct their clinical experience and to understand the complexity of their work in vastly different clinical settings, but on the other, they reflect the social and experimental reality of the individual and thus become subjective and often personal documents.
>
> (Wenzel *et al.* 1998).

The individual approach to reflection, which is ultimately about personal growth and development, is limited in its social contextual consideration and also lacks an overt action perspective (Barnett 1997).

Similarly, one study revealed that academics noted that, when receiving student reflections for assessment purposes, they were fully aware, and indeed concerned, that the students weren't presenting the full picture: 'academics initially expressed concern that some of the narratives submitted for assessment were a representation of only the students' perceived clinical competence with minimal description of the problems, dilemmas and "messiness" inherent in clinical practice' (Levett-Jones 2007). One way of reducing this effect is to provide support and guidance for you as a nursing student. Students report that they want and need support for their reflections and value this when the mentor or clinical placement coordinator takes the time to do so (O'Donovan 2006). Interestingly the university lecturer is viewed by students in some cases as having a minimal role in this (O'Donovan 2006). Without this support and guidance, situations are left open to multiple interpretations by students, and although there is value in personal reflection, it can often focus solely on students' particular views on events and what they might do differently the next time.

Activity 5

If you have used a model of reflection, such as outlined in Activity 4, within the context of professional nursing in your Nursing School, consider whether you believe your use of this led to personal development?

Do you believe, looking back, that it prompted reflection most concerned with you and your feelings, or did it encourage you to look beyond your own experiences and emotions and consider the environment within which the episode took place?

Do you believe that your reflections on nursing practice ought ultimately to shape and develop practice in some way, rather than merely be self-development?

Write your answers down before proceeding with the chapter.

While Schön originally described a model of reflection in and on action, this was primarily for qualified practitioners who would have practice knowledge upon which to base interpretations. A student may not have this particular knowledge so is rather going it alone in many regards. This personalized approach may encourage the student to focus on the 'me' rather than the 'me in the world'. Using a *critical* approach would consider the wider context. Furthermore, this focus on individuals and their personal feelings may be the cause of reluctance among some students to engage in self-reflection (Joyce 2005). Student reluctance to reveal innermost thoughts and feelings within reflection has been reported and it is a source of anxiety (Mitchell 1994). As the ultimate aim of a student portfolio is learning, based on a collection of a variety of evidence, mere personalized self-reflection for personal self-development appears inadequate to fully interpret the meaning and extract relevant learning from the portfolio journey (Boud *et al.* 1985: 10). Without consideration of models of reflection that incorporate the wider social context, 'the portfolio, as a method of self-reflection, becomes a means to evaluate personal satisfaction and self-worth' (Wenzel *et al.* 1998). This seems to be a common theme throughout student portfolio use. While there is certainly some merit in self-development, and clearly a portfolio sub-aim is personal development, it is worth noting that the primary purpose of the portfolio is to display a cohesive account of work-based learning that contains relevant evidence from and critical reflection on practice. However, Klenowski (2002) believes that a portfolio provides students with a vehicle that can assist them to reflect on their own growth and development, and similarly Mitchell (1994) equates self-reflection within the portfolio with increased student confidence and self-awareness. There are currently many who view this approach to reflection as being of limited value, particularly in practice settings. The self-limited nature of many contemporary models of reflection used in nursing is further identified when comprehensiveness of content is taken into consideration.

> While Schön originally described a model of reflection in and on action this was primarily for qualified practitioners who would have practice knowledge upon which to base interpretations.

Comprehensiveness of content

Ronald Barnett, a Professor of Education at the Institute of Education, University of London, is highly critical of this personalized self-reflection for professional practice (Barnett 1997). Barnett suggests that it is limited in its scope and application. He is critical of the current use of self-reflection within disciplines, stating that it is often performed at a superficial level that he says can 'hardly be termed *critical* self-reflection' (Barnett 1997: 101; emphasis author's own). Furthermore, he suggests that the use of reflection *in* action, espoused in professional practices, lacks both effective action and sufficient theoretical context as it over-relies on personal reflection in the knowledge domain, thus paying little attention to the domain of the world in which the action takes place. In particular, he criticized Schön's (1983) narrow interpretation and application of reflection, which avoids the context of the wider world of practice. Although consideration of the world may seem over-ambitious, this does not refer to whole world, but rather the world as it applies to an individual. This may be a community of learning such as the class, or study group (Wenger *et al.* 2002) or a local area of practice such as the hospital ward (Høyrup and Elkjaer 2006: 39). Reflection thus needs to have a *critical* element, as Barnett suggests. Critical reflection is 'the questioning of contextual aspects that are taken-for-granted – social, cultural and political – within which the task is situated' (Høyrup 2004: 444). It also involves questioning of meanings of situations with regards to our roles and relationships (Høyrup 2004). Within student reflections, while personal learning is important, ascribing meaning to these within the relevant context and associated with particular knowledge of a discipline has particular relevance for the overall aims of the portfolio. (Høyrup 2004: 444) argues that while reflection can result in new knowledge, critical reflection: 'may imply changes in the very psychological mechanisms that constitute the basis of our interpretations of the world'. Boud *et al.* (2006) concur with Barnett's views, suggesting that: 'reflection must be rethought and recontextualised so that it can fit more appropriately within group settings. It must also shift from its origins in concerns about individuals to learning within organizations' (Boud *et al.* 2006: 3a). In one chapter, 'Taking it beyond the individual', Høyrup and Elkjaer (2006: 29) further explore the limitations of the individual approach to reflection, suggesting instead the use of a 'critical perspective' that takes into account social, political and cultural influences, thus expanding the notion of reflection into critical reflection. Critical reflection involves a close examination of underpinning beliefs and values and a questioning of previously held assumptions (Høyrup and Elkjaer 2006).

> Reflection thus needs to have a critical element as Barnett (1997) suggests.

Critical reflection is further developed in a group of models based upon critical theory (Rolfe *et al.* 2001). These theoretical frameworks enable consideration of the wider influence of society (Mezirow 1983; Barnett 1997; Kim 1999; Taylor 2000; Taylor 2006). However, despite a commitment to critical theory, both Kim (1999) and Taylor (2000, 2006) lack the overt action perspective required within the operation of critical theory (Rolfe *et al.* 2001). Barnett (1997), on the other hand, is a very detailed and comprehensive model, grounded in critical theory, that provides explicit guidance aimed at critical reason, critical self-reflection and critical action.

In terms of origin, another point worth noting is that many of these models are concerned with analysis of *specific incidents* in practice rather than the comprehensive reflection that a portfolio may require. This use of 'critical incident' can be misleading for students who then seek adverse rather than ordinary situations to reflect upon. However, using a portfolio to reflect upon a critical incident has been reported in the literature (Hilliard 2006). Although Taylor's (2000, 2006) model drew directly from critical theory and refers to both contextual influences and an action imperative, the focus is largely upon the individual within discrete situations (Rolfe *et al.* 2001). Furthermore, while primarily concerned with specific incidents in practice, they also concur with Dewey's (1933) original notion of reflection emerging from a 'disturbance or uncertainty' (Høyrup and Elkjaer 2006:30). Thus the student begins the reflection with a problem or specific issue from the practice setting to reflect upon. Again, there is inconsistency here with the purposes of portfolio, whereby a specific incident is not in question but rather the need to reflect upon cumulative experience and products and processes of learning over time. Many individualized focused models of reflection are useful and valuable as tools for professional development (Taylor 2000, 2006; Rolfe *et al.* 2001; Rolfe 2005), yield valuable learning relevant for the practice situation (Kim 1999; Rolfe *et al.* 2001; Ekstrom 2002) and are often core components of contemporary portfolio development (Moon 1999; McMullan *et al.* 2003). However, consideration of the origin of reflection reveals the inherent nonconformity with the aims of a portfolio, which requires a systematic, detailed framework that examines the products and processes of learning in order to apply meaning and ultimately learn from this journey.

> In terms of origin, another point worth noting is that many of these models are concerned with analysis of specific incidents in practice rather than the comprehensive reflection that a portfolio may require.

You as a student require an all-encompassing model within your portfolio that not only provides the critical perspective required but also moves towards the 'organisational perspective' described by Høyrup and Elkjaer (2006: 39). Your portfolio takes place within the domain of practice rather than an individual context. Barnett (1997) appears to be the only model examined that moves beyond the individual to provide both the critical theory and organization perspective required within a comprehensive framework for critical reason, critical self-reflection and critical action. Barnett (1997) is less widely used in nursing and allied health literature (1 per cent citation in the literature search); however, he is widely cited in educational literature. A search of the Educational Resources Information Centre (ERIC) revealed 124 citations.

Barnett (1997) appears to be the only model examined that moves beyond the individual to provide both the critical theory and organization perspective required within a comprehensive framework for critical reason, critical self-reflection and critical action.

Another trend within the literature is the use of reflection within the context of teaching and learning. Gibbs (1988) provides a simplistic model that is useful for education within the classroom, and although widely used by nursing students, and often in portfolios (Pearce 2003), it may not be fully suited to the aims of a portfolio for the reasons already discussed. It is individualistic focused, has a verbalist orientation and has undergone little testing or development in the practice setting. Jasper (2006a: 68) suggests that this is a 'micro' approach to reflection that can be carried around in 'a mental framework for reflection on action'. Gibbs' framework is also thought to be 'a generalised educational framework and therefore is not focused on practice' (Jasper 2003). At the same time, Boud and Walker (1990, 1993) present a new perspective on educative reflection termed learning from experience.

Some models of reflection have a verbalist orientation and serve as a 'micro' approach to reflection that can be carried around in 'a mental framework for reflection on action'.

Indeed, Boud et al. (2006) specifically refer to *workplace learning* in a recent text. Boud et al. (1985) initially describe a model of reflection designed for students to learn from experience. This original model is referred to in 12 per cent of papers in the literature search. Interestingly, although a lot of development has occurred since the original paper there were no references within the search to any of this latter work (Boud and Walker 1990, 1993; Andresen et al. 2000; Boud et al. 2006). The aims of a portfolio are ultimately to uncover learning from reflection upon products and processes; for this purpose, many of the reflective frameworks currently in use are inapt. From an analysis of origins, two frameworks emerge as useful: Boud and Walker (1990, 1993) and Barnett (1997). A hybrid of these two frameworks has potential for use within a portfolio. This suggested framework emerges from an analysis of the origins of reflection. This will be further discussed in Chapter 6.

> From an analysis of origins two frameworks emerge as useful: Boud and Walker (1990, 1993) and Barnett (1997).

The portfolio aims to develop your knowledge as a student. This knowledge development, as described in Chapter 1, ultimately takes place within communities of practice, and is not merely the responsibility of an individual. Hence the rationale to consider more far-reaching models of reflection. These will be considered in more detail in Chapter 6. Consideration must be given to the choice of frameworks or models used within the reflective element of the portfolio in addition to the overarching framework that may be used. It may be useful to have a variety of theoretical frameworks. It is important for the user to be cognizant that frameworks and models are just that; they are not linear or prescriptive and can be used merely to facilitate a learning experience. Common to all models of reflection is reflective writing and the issues associated with this will now be described.

Reflective writing

Writing is a purposeful activity that is a means of communication. It is a way of ordering thoughts; it helps to release hitherto unexamined thoughts and helps to focus mental activity and facilitate creativity (Jasper 2006b). Reflective writing is a particular form of writing that is performed for the purposes of learning (Jasper 2006b). It allows for deep and complex understanding of a subject or experience (Jasper 2006b). Reflective writing can be categorized within two main domains: analytical and creative. Analytical writing involves analysing situations using a structured approach whereas creative writing is freer including activities such as story telling, poetry or keeping a journal. Typically within the portfolio the analytical writing required is guided by the chosen model of reflection, although creative approaches are sometimes employed (Hull *et al.* 2005). One difficulty when employing analytical writing techniques is the need to be less descriptive and more reflective, which students in Shields's (1995) study quickly realized.

Activity 6

Write one or two pages on your last experience on public transport before proceeding with the chapter.

Jasper (2006b) provides a very good chapter on reflective writing. She highlights the importance of reflective writing 'to provide evidence to demonstrate our continuing developing competence as practitioners' (Jasper 2006b: 81), although she observes that students often find it difficult to start this writing. Did you find it difficult to start writing for Activity 6? She suggests that when writing about practice it should be triggered by an experience that stands out. This could be an issue from practice that is on your mind, or a situation where you feel your knowledge could be improved, or a situation from practice that gives you particular satisfaction. It is also worth noting that it can be time-consuming so it is best to set aside time for this activity. Were you rushed completing Activity 6? And did this affect your ability to complete this task? Consider these barriers to writing when you are expected to write for your portfolio. Shields (1995) notes that while students are initially reticent about reflective writing, they adapt quickly with facilitation, and that this is also true for qualified nurses. They initially felt that while reflective thoughts were natural, reflective writing was not (Shields 1995).

When writing about practice Jasper (2006a) suggests that it should be triggered by an experience that stands out. This could be an issue from practice that is on your mind or a situation where you feel your knowledge could be improved, or a situation from practice that gives you particular satisfaction.

Students often have difficulty writing more than superficial and unconnected comments within reflective writing (Serembus 2000), therefore the provision of facilitation and support for reflection is a useful adjunct to student support. You might find that this is a particular issue for you. As reflective writing is a self-directed activity, as described in Chapter 1, facilitation ought to be a key component of this independent learning. Although this has time and resource issues for both teachers and staff in the clinical area (and, of course, you as a student), it is a useful and worthwhile activity that can enrich your learning from reflection. Interestingly:

- students often struggle with portfolios where there is lack of preparation and guidance;
- they view mentor support as crucial;

- Clinical Placement Coordinators have been identified as a very useful support;
- time can be a negating factor and the level of support to individuals varies according to individual nurses' commitments and motivation.

(O'Donovan 2006)

A further barrier to this support is lack of staff familiarity with the concept of reflection, thus creating a lack of confidence. This may be easily rectified by local information sessions and the use of clear guidelines on the topic. Similarly this can be an issue for students who report confusion about the use of reflection when formal teaching on the topic is received (Turner and Beddoes 2007).

Activity 7

If you are engaged in reflective writing in clinical practice, think about the support that you would like or require. Write down some ideas.

Can you identify barriers to reflective writing in yourself? In the practice environment?

Consider ways in which these barriers may be reduced.

Procrastination is common, with students reporting much thinking about portfolio reflection but little writing (Cayne 1997). Indeed, Nagayda and her colleagues (Nagayda *et al.* 2005) devote a whole chapter in their book on professional portfolios in occupational therapy to this very topic, entitled 'overcoming procrastination'. Students may be facilitated in their reflections while either attending clinical practice areas or within the classroom setting. Planning class time to facilitate students' progress, provide individual and group discussion and offer feedback have been offered as practical suggestions to overcome some of the difficulties that students face (Serembus 2000). Nurses in Jasper's (1999) study suggested that reflective writing needed a commitment and personal motivation. In her interviews with these qualified nurses it was revealed that the process of reflective writing required within a portfolio developed an ability for analytical writing and reflective skills (Jasper 1999). The writing also was a learning in itself that helped personal development (Jasper 1999).

It is important for both teachers and students to take cognizance of the issues that surround facilitated reflection such as confidentiality, credibility and honesty. Clear guidelines regarding these issues also need to be in place in addition to a pathway for disclosure should students reveal items during reflective writing or discussions that may warrant reporting within the health service or elsewhere. These guidelines ought to be developed locally in a partnership arrangement with health service providers. Although it is beyond the remit of this book to consider all the practice issues that may arise as a result of student reflection, some brief guidelines in relation to ethical and legal issues are provided at the end of the chapter.

There is very little by way of example within the literature about reflective writing. One medical journal, *Academic Emergency Medicine*, features some descriptions of incidents in practice recorded by junior doctors as portfolio entries (Chisholm and Croskerry 2004; Walthall *et al.* 2006). These give some guidance on generalized reflective writing in terms of description of events. However, they appear to lack a reflective approach. They reveal negative feelings towards clients, and display the limitation of the individualistic/personal reflection. The whole discussion is focused on the self in the situation, with neither consideration of the context in which the two incidents took place nor any reference to research or literature on the topic that might enhance personal interpretation. Ultimately there is little by way of implications for practice and perhaps some ethical issues that are yet unaddressed.

Recently an example of a nursing student's reflective narrative has been provided (Levett-Jones 2007). This author reveals that having a narrative that may be read by faculty staff is a barrier to student expression (Levett-Jones 2007). Again, the narrative isn't particularly critical and is focused mostly on the self, a point reiterated by the lecturers involved in marking, who were concerned that the full realities of the practice situations were not being revealed within student narratives. One drawback with this suggested use of narrative is the simplistic verbalist framework supplied (What happened? So what? Now what?). Therefore the use of a more rigorous framework may guide student reflective writing more appropriately. Furthermore, the use of this particular model encourages students to focus on a clinical 'episode', leading them to consider and look for unusual incidents in practice rather than the ordinary. A similar approach is also advocated by Jasper (2006b: 85), suggesting reflective writing on 'the witnessing of poor professional practice . . . [or] . . . difficulties within interpersonal relationships'. While there may be some merit in this approach it is less consistent with the modern interpretation of critical reflection; furthermore, in the absence of rigorous frameworks for reflection and appropriate support and reporting mechanisms for students there is an associated risk in terms of ethical issues, which will be discussed later. Interestingly, some nurses in Shields's study, while reporting reflection as a valuable tool for professional development, viewed reflection as 'dangerous in unskilled or unsupervised hands' (Shields 1995).

The nature and type of reflective writing will be guided to a certain extent by the chosen model of reflection. However Hull *et al.* (2005) provide useful guidelines on commencing this writing (Table 3.1).

Hull *et al.* (2005) indicate the importance of client confidentiality, so this and other ethical issues associated with reflection and reflective writing will now be briefly considered.

Table 3.1 Guidelines on commencing reflective writing

- Be frank and honest in your entries.
- Be open and sincere.
- Have a positive approach.
- Be spontaneous, don't spend a lot of time working out what it is you are going to write.
- Express yourself in other ways, using diagrams, pictures, poetry.
- Ensure client confidentiality.

Source: Hull *et al.* (2005).

Ethical and legal issues

While there is a great deal of literature pertaining to the use of portfolios within nurse education, little by way of guidance or research exists regarding the management of ethical issues (Howarth 1999). As the use of reflective writing commits the student's views to paper it may be a cause of concern to many nurse educators because of the potential professional, legal, moral and ethical issues that may arise (Burns and Bulman 2000). Hargreaves (1997) suggests that any discussion of patient care outside the clinical area for the purpose of reflection requires a 'code of ethics'. Burns and Bulman (2000) suggest that informed consent should be gained from the client where reflective writing is planned; this is not always a legal requirement for students once absolute confidentiality is maintained.

The origins of reflection as discussed earlier in the chapter reveal a historical orientation towards reflecting on specific incidents that occur in practice, which in many ways still influences the use of many models of reflection even if they do not specify the nature of the event to be reflected upon. This legacy is evident in Jasper's (2006b) suggestions for nurses' reflective writing, calling upon them to examine areas that bother them in practice, or that they cannot get off their mind. This list includes witnessing of poor practice and interpersonal conflict (Jasper 2006b). All documents may, however, be potentially discoverable through an order of the courts, and this equally applies to reflective writing. This highlights the facilitator's responsibility to take appropriate action if incidences of concern emerge through these reflective writings. Failure to act in these cases could result in the educator being found negligent or a party to the act. These issues may be dealt with in local guidelines on portfolios and reflective writing depending on the particular regulations governing the country and the professional bodies concerned. Furthermore, direction may be given within portfolio guidelines with regard to appropriate use of critical incidents. Benner's (2000) identification of critical incidents in nursing, although primarily designed for qualified staff, is perhaps more in keeping with the spirit of the portfolio and its ultimate aim of learning and knowledge development, and may prevent students from inadvertently relying on reflective writing as a mechanism for reporting incidents which may be best reported using appropriate means (Table 3.2).

In keeping with Hargreaves's (1997) suggestion of a code of ethics to guide reflective writing, it may be useful to consider the ethical principles that may apply. Ethics refers to the study of morals and relates to the issues of right and wrong in the theory and practice of human behaviour. It is a set of principles used to guide researchers. There are four main principles often used to guide researchers: respect for autonomy, nonmaleficence, beneficence and justice. Autonomy respects people's right to make free choices about their own lives. This means that a client chooses freely whether to participate or not and to have full knowledge about what the involvement entails (Burns and Bulman 2000). It may be that where a specific client is required for the reflective writing, such as a case study, informed consent is obtained from participants (Burns and Bulman 2000). Within this context confidentiality and anonymity must also be preserved, and this is one aspect that is highlighted within the literature (Jasper 2006b; Hull *et al.* 2005).

Nonmaleficence means the duty of not inflicting harm on another person. The possibility of physical, psychological, social and personal harm being caused to an individual during research studies must always be prevented. In a similar way, reflective writing must not harm the student, staff or client involved. A client could be harmed through breaking anonymity and confidentiality, as outlined above. Similarly, a staff member whose actions are described could be potentially harmed through this. From the student's perspective the harm may not be immediately obvious. However, if the reflective writing, particularly in the absence of supervision or facilitation, serves as a means of complaint about a particular issue, then the student is inadvertently deprived of the appropriate mechanism wherein to raise the complaint. In addition, reflective writing may raise personal issues that perhaps neither the preceptor/mentor nor the student are able to deal with and there could be, in absence of clear guidelines and provisions, little by way of structured support, such as counselling, for these emotional issues. Hargreaves (1997), in her discussion of the ethical issues associated with using reflection in nurse education settings, refers to this latter issue as student vulnerability.

Beneficence builds on the principle of nonmaleficence and concerns the promotion of good. Ultimately nurses and nursing students aim to provide

Table 3.2 Benner's categories for critical incidents in nursing

- Those in which interventions really made a difference.
- Those that went unusually well.
- Those in which there was a breakdown.
- Those that were ordinary and typical.
- Those that captured the essence of nursing.
- Those that were particularly demanding.

Source: Benner (2000).

the best care to clients and to strive constantly to improve that care. Any threat to client anonymity could threaten this. If the student or nurse emerges as vulnerable as a result of a student reflection, ultimately the experience may not be entailing the promotion of good. From an ethical perspective one would expect the portfolio and reflections within the portfolio ultimately to benefit the student in terms of knowledge development.

While Hargreaves (1997) argues that challenging status quo in nursing may go hand in hand with reflection, there is nothing to suggest within the literature that reflection, or reflective writing, are the appropriate mechanisms for doing so. This further potentiates the vulnerability of students who are perhaps lured to an unreliable system of reporting incidents.

Although it is you as a student that completes the portfolio, the Nursing School or the educational establishment may incur a certain responsibility for the portfolio contents (Pearce 2003). A document becoming the subject of a legal discovery or written reports of bad practice could be interpreted as the student's 'reporting' of this matter (Pearce 2003). These are obviously complex legal matters, but it is possible that extreme freedom in the use of the portfolio that is pertaining to its use in the widest sense of the interpretation of collection of evidence leaves room for potential problems (Pearce 2003). As with Endacott's (Endacott et al. 2004) findings, Nursing Schools as they establish further are beginning to place more stringent guidelines that ensure more appropriate use of both the portfolio and the reflective writing. These include clear guidelines for portfolio use, the use of facilitation to guide reflection and reflective writing and the development of ethical guidelines for use therein.

Conclusion

Reflection, and specifically critical reflection, is an inherent component of portfolio use. This moves beyond personal introspection and personal development to consider the wider influences on practice and framing learning within this context. From an analysis of the origins of reflection, consideration and development of models of reflection that are particularly suited to educational environments is limited. So too are the popular approaches to reflection in nursing which focus on personal and professional development rather than a broader concept of knowledge development. Popular contemporary models that focus on critical practice and learning from experience, although not used extensively within nursing, are proposed as possible alternatives for use. Reflective writing forms an important component of reflection within the portfolio although guidelines on this area are sparse. Current literature suggests several tips for getting started (Jasper 2006b) and operating within Benner's (2000) categories may be a useful guide for appropriation of writing. Consideration needs also to be given to legal and ethical parameters within which this writing takes place and, as with all stages of the portfolio, facilitation is key to success in this area.

Summary of key points

- Reflection is an inherent component of portfolio use.
- Reflection in nursing has its roots in the seminal work of Dewey, Kolb and Schön.
- Some models of reflection were developed specifically for professional development, others for educational purposes.
- Reflective writing forms an important component of reflection within the portfolio. This can be difficult to start and needs time set aside. It is useful to think of a subject or experience that interested or surprised you.

Recommended further reading

Barnett, R. (1997) *Higher Education: A Critical Business*. Bristol: Society for Research into Higher Education.
Jasper, M. (2003) *Beginning Reflective Practice: Foundations in Nursing and Health Care*. Cheltenham: Nelson Thornes.
Rolfe, G., Freshwater, D. *et al.* (2001) *Critical Reflection for Nursing and the Helping Professions: A User's Guide*. Basingstoke: Palgrave.

References

Andresen, L., Boud, D. *et al.* (2000) Experience based learning, in G. Foley (ed.) *Understanding Adult Education and Training*. Sydney: Allen & Unwin.
Barnett, R. (1997) *Higher Education: A Critical Business*. Buckingham: Open University Press/Taylor and Francis.
Benner, P. D. (2000) *From Novice to Expert: Excellence and Power in Clinical Nursing Practice*, Commemorative Edition. New Jersey: Prentice Hall.
Boud, D., Cressey, P. *et al.* (2006) Setting the scene for productive reflection at work, in D. Boud, P. Cressey and P. Doherty (eds) *Productive Reflection at Work*. Oxford: Routledge.
Boud, D., Keogh, R. *et al.* (1985) Promoting reflection in learning: a model, in D. Boud, D. Walker and R. Keogh (eds) *Reflection: Turning Experience into Learning*. London: Kogan Page.
Boud, D. and Walker, D. (1990) Making the most of experience, *Studies in Continuing Education*, 12(2): 61–80.

Boud, D. and Walker, D. (1993) Barriers to reflection on experience, in D. Boud, R. Cohen and D. Walker (eds) *Using Experience For Learning*. Buckingham: Society for Research into Higher Education and Open University Press.

Brackenreg, J. (2004) Issues in reflection and debriefing: how nurse educators structure experiential activities, *Nurse Education in Practice*, 4(4): 264–70.

Burns, S. and Bulman, C. (2000) *Reflective Practice in Nursing: The Growth of the Professional Practitioner*. Oxford: Blackwell Science.

Calhoun, C. J. (1995) *Critical Social Theory: Culture, History, and the Challenge of Difference*. Oxford: Blackwell Publishing.

Carper, B. A. (1978) Fundamental patterns of knowing in nursing, *Advanced Nursing Science*, 1(1): 13–23.

Carroll, M., Curtis, L. *et al.* (2002) Is there a place for reflective practice in the nursing curriculum?, *Nurse Education in Practice*, 2(1): 13–20.

Cayne, J. V. (1997) Portfolios: a developmental influence?, in P. Abbott and R. Sapsford (eds), *Research into Practice: A Reader*. Buckingham: Open University Press.

Chisholm, C. D. and Croskerry, P. (2004) A case study in medical error: the use of the portfolio entry, *Academic Emergency Medicine*, 11(4): 388–92.

Dewey, J. (1933) *How We Think: A Restatement of the Relation of Reflective Thinking to the Educative Process*. Boston: Heath and Co.

Ekstrom, D. N. (2002) An international collaboration in nursing education viewed through the lens of critical social theory, *Journal of Nursing Education*, 41(7): 289–94.

Endacott, R., Gray, M. A. *et al.* (2004) Using portfolios in the assessment of learning and competence: the impact of four models, *Nurse Education in Practice*, 4(4): 250–7.

English National Board for Nurses, Midwives and Health Visitors (1994) *Creating Lifelong Learners: Partnerships for Care*. London: ENBNMHV.

Fawcett, J. (1995) *Analysis and Evaluation of Conceptual Models of Nursing*, 3rd edn. Philadelphia, PA: F.A. Davies.

Gibbs, G. (1988) *Learning by Doing: A Guide to Teaching Learning Methods*. Oxford: Oxford Brookes University.

Habermas, J. (1971) *Knowledge and Human Interests*. Boston: Beacon Press.

Hargreaves, J. (1997) Using patients: exploring the ethical dimension of reflective practice in nurse education, *Journal of Advanced Nursing*, 25(2): 223–8.

Held, D. (1980) *Introduction to Critical Theory: Horkheimer to Habermas*. Los Angeles, CA: University of California Press.

Hilliard, C. (2006) Using structured reflection on a critical incident to develop a professional portfolio, *Nursing Standard*, 21(2): 35–40.

How, A. (2003) *Critical Theory*. Basingstoke: Palgrave Macmillan.

Howarth, A. (1999) Education: the portfolio as an assessment tool in midwifery education, *British Journal of Midwifery*, 7: 327–9.

Høyrup, S. (2004) Reflection as a core process in organisational learning, *The Journal of Workplace Learning*, 16(8): 442–54.

Høyrup, S. and Elkjaer, B. (2006) Reflection: taking it beyond the individual, in D. Boud, P. Cressey and P. Doherty (eds) *Productive Reflection at Work*. Oxford: Routledge.

Hull, C., Redfern, J. *et al.* (2005) *Profiles and Portfolios: A Guide for Health and Social Care*. Basingstoke: Palgrave Macmillan.

Hull, C. and Redfern, L. (1996) *Profiles and Portfolios: A Guide for Nurses and Midwives*. Basingstoke: Macmillan.

Jarvis, P. (1992) Reflective practice and nursing, *Nurse Education Today*, 12(3): 174–81.

Jasper, M. (2003) *Beginning Reflective Practice: Foundations in Nursing and Health Care.* Cheltenham: Nelson Thornes.

Jasper, M. A. (1999) Nurses'perceptions of the value of written reflection, *Nurse Education Today*, 19(6): 452–63.

Jasper, M. (2006a) Reflection and reflective practice, in M. Jasper (ed.) *Professional Development, Reflection and Decision Making*, pp 39–80, Oxford: Blackwell Publishing.

Jasper, M. (2006b) Reflective writing for professional development, in M. Jasper (ed.) *Professional Development, Reflection and Decision Making*, pp 81–106, Oxford: Blackwell Publishing.

Jasper, M. (2006c) Portfolios and the use of evidence, in M. Jasper (ed.) *Professional Development, Reflection and Decision Making*. Oxford: Blackwell Publishing.

Johns, C. ([1999] 2004) *Becoming a Reflective Practitioner*, pp 154–183, Oxford: Blackwell.

Joyce, P. (2005) A framework for portfolio development in postgraduate nursing practice, *Journal of Clinical Nursing*, 14(4): 456–63.

Kim, H. S. (1999) Critical reflective inquiry for knowledge development in nursing practice, *Journal of Advanced Nursing*, 29(5): 1205–12.

Klenowski, V. (2002) *Developing Portfolios for Learning and Assessment: Processes and Principles*. Oxford: Routledge.

Kolb, D. A. (1984) *Experimental Learning*. London: Prentice Hall.

Levett-Jones, T. L. (2007) Facilitating reflective practice and self-assessment of competence through the use of narratives, *Nurse Education in Practice*, 7(2): 112–19.

Lyons, N. (1998) *With Portfolio in Hand: Validating the New Teacher Professionalism.* New York: Teachers College Press.

Mackintosh, C. (1998) Reflection: a flawed strategy for the nursing profession, *Nurse Education Today*, 18(7): 553–7.

McMullan, M., Endacott, R. *et al.* (2003) Portfolios and assessment of competence: a review of the literature, *Journal of Advanced Nursing*, 41(3): 283–94.

Mezirow, J. (1983) A critical theory of adult learning and education, in M. Tight (ed.) *Education for Adults: Educational Opportunities for Adults*. Beckenham: Croom Helm in association with the Open University.

Mitchell, M. (1994) The views of students and teachers on the use of portfolios as a learning and assessment tool in midwifery education, *Nurse Education Today*, 14(1): 38–43.

Moon, J. A. (1999) *Learning Journals: A Handbook for Academics, Students and Professional Development*. London: Kogan Page.

Nagayda, J., Schindehette, S. *et al.* (2005) *The Professional Portfolio in Occupational Therapy Career Development and Continuing Competence*. Thorofare, NJ: Slack Incorporated.

National Health Service Management Executive (1993) *A Vision for the Future*. London: Department of Health.

O'Donovan, M. (2006) Reflecting during clinical placement: discovering factors that influence pre-registration psychiatric nursing students, *Nurse Education in Practice*, 6(3): 134–40.

Pearce, R. (2003) *Profiles and Portfolios of Evidence*. Cheltenham: Nelson Thornes.

Rolfe, G. (2005) The deconstructing angel: nursing, reflection and evidence-based practice, *Nursing Inquiry*, 12(2): 78–86.

Rolfe, G., Freshwater, D. *et al.* (2001) *Critical Reflection for Nursing and the Helping Professions: A User's Guide*, Basingstoke: Palgrave.

Schön, D. A. (1983) *The Reflective Practitioner*. New York: Basic Books.

Serembus, J. F. (2000) Teaching the process of developing a professional portfolio, *Nurse Educator*, 25(6): 282–7.

Shields, E. (1995) Reflection and learning in student nurses, *Nurse Education Today*, 15(452): 8.

Taylor, B. (2000) *Reflective Practice: A Guide for Nurses and Midwives*. Buckingham: Open University Press.

Taylor, B. (2006) *Reflective Practice: a Guide for Nurses and Midwives*, 2nd edn. Buckingham: Open University Press.

Teekman, B. (2000) Exploring reflective thinking in nursing practice, *Journal of Advanced Nursing*, 31(5): 1125–35.

Turner, D. S. and Beddoes, L. (2007) Using reflective models to enhance learning: experiences of staff and students, *Nurse Education in Practice*, 7(3): 135–40.

UKCC (1996) PREP and profiling. *Register*, 17: 7–10.

Walthall, J., Martin, M. L. *et al.* (2006) Resident portfolio: Dr. death – reflections of death telling . . . including commentary by Marco CA, *Academic Emergency Medicine*, 13(4): 462.

Wenger, E. C., Mc Dermott, R. *et al.* (2002) *Cultivating Communities of Practice: A Guide to Managing Knowledge*. Boston, MA: Harvard Business School Press.

Wenzel, L. S., Briggs, K. L. *et al.* (1998) Portfolio: authentic assessment in the age of the curriculum revolution, *Journal of Nursing Education*, 37(5): 209–12.

4

Competence in Nursing

Miriam Farrell and Fiona Timmins

*Introduction • What is competence? • Assessment of competence •
Assessment of competence using portfolios • Conclusion • Summary of key
points • Recommended further reading • References*

Introduction

In addition to supporting the integration of classroom teaching and practical
experiences in nursing, portfolios are also used as a method to support a
measure of competence (Garrett and Jackson 2006). It is possible that you are
familiar with a system such as this, where the portfolio forms part of the measurement of your competency in the clinical nursing environment. It may be
that you present some of the evidence from the portfolio to show that you are
competent at a particular aspect of nursing practice. Before dealing with the
interface between the portfolio and competence it is worth considering our
understanding of the term competence. Much of the literature on competence
reveals it to be an important factor in student learning and assessment in the
United Kingdom (UK), United States of America (USA) and Australia. Clinical
competence assessment now forms a large component of students' overall
assessment within preparatory nurse education programmes. The transition to
competence-based approaches from more traditional approaches has influenced the introduction of a variety of assessment tools. The majority of
research on the topic originates in the UK (Calman *et al.* 2002; Watson *et al.*

2002; Dolan 2003) and this will be utilized to inform the development of our understanding in this area.

Activity 1

Whether or not you are familiar with the term competence, consider its meaning within the context of student learning within nursing practice.

Write down your observations before proceeding with the chapter.

Remember!

Competence assessment is an important concept in contemporary approaches to nurse education. The measurement of competence, as opposed to more traditionally and possibly subjective approaches, requires the use of specific assessment tools, of which there are many.

What is competence?

The concept of clinical competence arose in North America and is not unique to the profession of nursing (Calman *et al.* 2002). However, in a comprehensive systematic review of the research on clinical competence literature emerging between 1980 and 2000, Watson *et al.* (2002) suggest that the use of competence approaches within nurse education, despite the lack of novelty with its use internationally, in some cases failed to respond to potential pitfalls or challenges that may have been identified in the literature by others who had gone down this road before. Despite this, Watson *et al.* conclude that competence-based approaches for assessment of nursing student performance in clinical practice settings are useful.

The nursing literature is replete with discussions from the UK, USA and Australia regarding the complexity of competence and the broad spectrum of ways in which competence can be defined, operationalized and assessed (Ashworth and Morrison 1991; Girot 1993; Bradshaw 1997; Chambers 1998; Eraut 1998; Milligan 1998; Storey 2001). It appears that the confusion surrounding the definition of competence, however, is not unique to pre-registration nursing but also applies to specialist and advanced practice in nursing and midwifery (Worth-Butler *et al.* 1996; Cattini and Knowles 1999; Dunn *et al.* 2000). The *Concise Oxford English Dictionary* (Urdang 1992) describes 'competent' as being adequately qualified, capable or effective and 'competence' as the state of being competent. The terms competence, competency and competencies are used interchangeably within the literature with no consensus on term use emerging. Watson *et al.* suggest difficulty with the reliability and validity of competence assessment tools, and different understanding of the term competence can compound this problem. Suppose, for example, you are being assessed by a nurse with regard to your competence in one proficiency outlined by the National Nursing Council (NMC 2004): developing professional and ethical practice. The nurse's understanding of the term competence may affect the ultimate judgement of whether you are deemed competent or not. This openness to interpretation (if it is present) is an example of something that can affect the *validity and reliability* of the tool. Validity refers to the ability of the assessment to measure what it says it measures, and reliability relates to the consistency of the findings over time. Would the assessment yield the same or similar results one week from now? One simple way of increasing the validity of the measure, of course, is to develop a common and consistent understanding of the concept that is being measured – competence; however, this too can be problematic.

Activity 2

Is the term 'competence' familiar to you in relation to your own assessments within nursing practice?

If this term is in use (without looking at your documentation), write down what it means to you.

Now examine whether a definition, description or outline of elements of competence is in use within your Nursing School. Is it obvious from your documentation? How does it compare to your own description and understanding of the term?

Write down your observations before proceeding with the chapter.

Storey and Haigh (2002) suggest that while there is no common approach or agreed definition of competence, emerging competency definitions combine three main categories: what students should be like; attributes students need to possess and what students need to achieve. However, competence is further conceptualized as comprising three main approaches: first, behaviourist, whereby the performance of a specified behaviour or task may be observed and measured. Secondly, there is reference to generic competence pertaining to a cluster of generalized abilities of the student and, finally, holistic approaches, which include cognitive, psychomotor and affective domains of learning (Gonczi 1999; Sinclair and Gardner 1999; Dunn *et al.* 2000; Watkins 2000; Ramritu and Barnard 2001; Zhang *et al.* 2001; Griffith *et al.* 2002). While a plethora of literature exists on the subject, much of the work is anecdotal, discussion or management papers with some empirical studies emerging. This means that when your teachers are attempting to find an evidence-based approach to the development of their understanding of competence, this can be hampered by a lack of detailed study on the topic, although expert opinion does exist. The use of behaviourist approaches to competence has been reported, and Dolan (2003) revealed that students felt their placements were dominated by the achievement of individual competencies, inhibiting their gaining of a holistic experience of care. This finding is consistent with previous studies (Worth-Butler *et al.* 1996; Ramritu and Barnard 2001) on the topic, and an opinion is being formed that a holistic approach to the development of competence is the way forward for nursing students, which is echoed in smaller qualitative studies (Girot 1993; Ramritu and Barnard 2001).

Competency definitions combine three main categories:

- What students should be like.
- Attributes students need to possess.
- What students need to achieve.

Approaches to competence are further described:

Behaviourist: necessitating the performance of a specified behaviour or task that can be observed or measured.

Generic: referring to a cluster of generalized abilities.

Holistic: includes a mix of approaches such as cognitive, psychomotor and affective.

Although contemporary approaches ultimately aim for a consistent, objective, rigorous approach to the assessment of student performance in the clinical area, competence and competence-based approaches are inherently complex. This discussion of competence highlights some of the atomized views and approaches to competence development that appear to conflict with gaining a holistic understanding and experience of care and development of competence.

Assessment of competence

The assessment of nursing student performance in clinical practice has always been a challenging aspect of pre-registration education. Over the years a number of approaches have been adopted: assessments in the practical room during the 1960s (which were criticized for being too far removed from real practice), replaced by ward-based practical assessments of key skills in the 1970s (which were judged to be too artificial and task-focused). These were in turn replaced by continuous assessment of clinical practice, which has continued in various forms since the 1980s (Watkins 2000). The move to continuous assessment has meant that education providers have had to design and apply assessment instruments to encompass the full range of pre-registration course outcomes. In addition, there is an increasing focus on the assessment of clinical competence in the UK since the advent of the publication *Making a Difference* (DoH 1999) and Fitness for Practice (UKCC 1999; Gannon *et al.* 2001).

Activity 3

Consider how you would best like to have your nursing skills assessed?

Research has long indicated that the clinical learning environment is the most influential context when considering the acquisition of nursing knowledge and skills. However, there is much criticism in the literature about clinical practice assessment that relates to concerns regarding the proliferation of poorly designed – and often untested – assessment instruments (Watson *et al.* 2002). Furthermore, a lack of consensus about the meaning of competence and its application to nursing (Bradshaw 1997, 1998; Eraut 1998; Watson *et al.* 2002) has contributed to continuing debate about how best to measure and assess clinical skills and how, for example, to distinguish between the competence of diploma and degree students. This debate occurs beyond the realm of the student, and does not indicate weakness in the system, but rather an open dialogue within a relatively new academic discipline. It is also consistent with debates in other disciplines and reflects the profession's desire for best practice and constantly seeking evidence to support practices.

The debate itself extends beyond assessment and has prompted a more fundamental challenge: that a competence-driven curriculum is antithetical to a higher education for nurses (Watson *et al.* 2002). In Australia it has been observed that 'the competency-based approach to nursing education is an indisputable reality but nursing competencies must not be allowed to control the curriculum' (Chapman 1999: 129).

Distinctions have been drawn between competence and performance to try to explain how the apparently competent nurse does not always perform to an adequate level (While 1994) and thus also to emphasize the importance of testing students in situations related as closely as possible to those of their future professional practice (Alinier 2003). In proposing a model of learning in which students know (knowledge), know how (competence), show how (performance) and do (action), it has been asserted that assessment procedures in nursing should aim to test the upper reaches of this hierarchy (Miller 1990). In a similar vein, Foster and Hawkins (2004) have proposed a 'performance of understanding' assessment model, which focuses on the application of knowledge in practice in both real and simulated situations, with the highest level of attainment indicated by evidence that the student gives a 'performance of understanding guided by tacit knowledge and reflexivity' (Foster and Hawkins 2004: 334). Perhaps not surprisingly, there appears to be a mismatch between these demanding expectations and the tools to measure clinical performance.

Queensland Nursing Council (2001) undertook a systematic review of the literature to identify indicators of competence for practice, to establish the effectiveness of the indicators in measuring competence to practise, and to summarize the best available evidence on methods of validation of the indicators. Their review draws attention to the continuing problems associated with the definition of competence and its measurement. They identified eight indicators commonly used in attempts to assess competence: continuing education, portfolios, examinations, peer review, direct observation, self-assessment, interviews and patient outcomes. The team was unable to identify any research to suggest that any one method was superior to the others, but perhaps more importantly, they noted that many papers they reviewed did not even mention issues of reliability and validity, and that where tools had been used to test validity they were generally complex. It is interesting that the portfolio emerges within this group as an indicator within competence assessment.

Indicators commonly used in attempts to assess competence (Queensland Nursing Council 2001)

- Continuing education
- Portfolios
- Examinations
- Peer review
- Direct observation
- Self-assessment
- Interviews
- Patient outcomes

This analysis has been confirmed by a more recent systematic review of the literature about clinical competence assessment (Watson *et al.* 2002). The review concluded that there is still considerable confusion about the definition of clinical competence, that most of the methods in use to define or measure competence have not been developed systematically, and that issues of reliability and validity have barely been addressed. In another evaluation of approaches to practice assessment, Shanley (2001) is explicit in his criticism of the inadequacy of the methods he reviewed, asserting that it could result in a loss of confidence in the profession's ability to safeguard the public.

Another systematic review of the literature addressing the measurement of nurse clinical performance draws attention to the continuing absence of universal approval for any particular instrument and to the diversity that continues to prevail (Robb *et al.* 2002). You may be aware of this if you have friends who are attending other Schools of Nursing, or working alongside students from another School; each of you may have quite different approaches and related documentation to support the assessment of your competence. Within nurse education there is a propensity towards continuous updating and development of necessary documentation. Acknowledging the continuing tendency to construct new instruments, Robb *et al.* suggest adoption of an approach to tool construction focusing on expected behaviours identified by experienced nurses reflecting on the requirements of their role (Robb *et al.* 2002). Others have reported on the use of the Delphi technique to develop and refine a clinical assessment tool (Lofmark and Wikblad 2001). This is where the opinions of experts/interested parties may be sought and confirmed over several rounds of refinement and development. However, these approaches perpetuate the system of local development that some commentators consider inappropriate and unlikely to involve the validity and reliability testing required.

The review by the Queensland Nursing Council (2001) predates an attempt in the UK to test selected competence tools for reliability and validity. Calman *et al.* (2002) undertook research in seven institutions in Scotland for the National Board. They compared items in selected assessment tools with statutory competencies for nurses and midwives by administering additional assessment measures. While the tools assessed showed good internal consistency, the non-specific nature of the (then UKCC) competencies meant that the approach to validity testing could not discriminate between more and less valid tools, raising doubts about sensitivity and ability to discriminate between competent and incompetent students. The team observed that very few students were failed on clinical grounds, suggesting bias or reluctance by practice assessors to judge students negatively, a tendency reinforced by Duffy's (2004) research. In their searching work on competence and performance assessment in the early 1990s, Fitzpatrick and colleagues found that observer training emerged as one of the most important strategies for addressing the potential for bias and error inherent in observational method (Fitzpatrick *et al.* 1996), the approach which remains the predominant method of clinical practice assessment.

One of the most striking findings arising from the research undertaken by

---

Activity 4

The literature indicates that the 'observation method' has potential inherent bias. Outline factors that could potentially contribute to bias on the part of the nurse in the assessment process.

Write down your observations.

Calman *et al.* (2002) was that none of the seven institutions in their study had carried out any tests to validate the assessment tools being used. They note that the diversity of tools they observed in use during their investigation sits uneasily with the requirement that all nurses and midwives in the UK are required to reach a national minimum level of competence. They claim that 'most tools used for assessing nursing and midwifery competence do not instil confidence in students or practice assessors, and practice assessors find them difficult to understand and apply to practice' (Calman *et al.* 2002). They conclude by arguing that there is a need for a national clinical competence tool so that minimum standards of competence of students on all pre-registration programmes can be assessed with confidence, making the point that such a tool could more readily be tested for reliability and validity than those developed locally.

Activity 5

If you are familiar with using an assessment tool are you confident with its ability to assess competence?

Write out three strengths of the tool.

Write out three areas of the tool that you believe require further development.

Write out your observations.

Confirmation of the continuing relevance of these proposals can be found in the review of the first *Fitness for Practice* schemes in England, which also concluded that national tools were required to establish a national competence assessment threshold (Scholes *et al.* 2004). Calman *et al.* (2002) further recommend and propose a robust training strategy for assessors, wider use of self-assessment by students, assessment of students by patients, and assessment of clinical tasks and procedures under simulated conditions using approaches such as the objective structured clinical examination (OSCE). In order to improve reliability and validity of current approaches to assessment, it is becoming increasingly clear that a comprehensive, well tested, nationally applied tool is something that needs serious consideration.

Competence-based approaches have also been criticized as being paper-driven, bureaucratic (Storey 2001) and time-consuming (Wilson-Barnett *et al.* 1995; Casey 2001; Griffin 2001), with problems noted in the language used in competency documentation (Neary 1999; Griffin 2001). These findings are supported in a recent study (Calman *et al.* 2002) in which students expressed the view that staff saw competence documentation as 'paperwork' and a 'tedious formality' rather than an integral part of their supervision and education. Do any of these findings concur with your views in Activity 5?

Increasingly portfolios are being use to support some approaches to competence assessment (Murrell *et al.* 1998; Griffin 2001). The use of a portfolio of evidence in conjunction with other forms of assessment may address some of the criticisms of competence assessment raised within the literature in terms of objectivity, and permits you as a student potentially to have an increased say in your overall assessment. It increases the range and scope of evidence that may be used to assess competence. Furthermore, it encourages a holistic approach rather than atomizing competence assessment into distinct items of work performance (Worth-Butler *et al.* 1996; Ramritu and Barnard 2001; Watson *et al.* 2002; Dolan 2003). It provides objective data towards competence assessment, that could easily be read later by a second assessor, unlike single observations of your practice by a nurse. That is not to say that a portfolio approach would replace observation, but rather contribute to a more holistic and possibly more objective and valid assessment method.

Remember!

The use of a portfolio to assess your competence can lead to a more holistic and objective approach to assessment.

Assessment of competence using portfolios

The portfolio is said to provide a means of developing your reflective abilities as a student and therefore competence development (Priest and Roberts 1998; McMullan *et al.* 2003; Hull *et al.* 2005). Indeed, the portfolio is often designed to measure 'acquisition and development of competence' (Jasper 2006). Two decades ago Benner (1984) linked reflection with the portfolio and competence development by suggesting that nurses examine the nature of nursing in personal portfolios, and continually identify the competencies that define nursing practice through reflective practice. More recently Lenburg (2000) extended this view by proposing that 'practice competence' could be improved by engaging in critical reflection and the use of a competence-based portfolio. Similarly, national publications in the Republic of Ireland have advocated the need to foster reflective skills within student nurses (Government of Republic of Ireland 1998; An Bord Altranais 2000). The call for reflection to remain an integral part of everyday practice is reiterated within modern approaches to nursing education that emphasize the acquisition of professional competencies through experience of, and reflection on practice in order to develop that practice (Government of Republic of Ireland 1998).

It is proposed that student participation and responsibility is enhanced through competence assessment where portfolios are used (Murrell *et al.* 1998; Griffin 2001; McMullan *et al.* 2003). The key to success is deemed to be the student's active engagement in the process (Murrell *et al.* 1998; Griffin 2001; McMullan *et al.* 2003). One study that aimed to identify links between variables believed to impact on clinical competence development revealed a relationship between the variable 'student effort' and 'clinical competence' (Baramee and Blegen 2003). It can be envisaged how student effort and responsibility could be impacted upon through the use of the portfolio within the competence assessment where students actively seek and provide evidence for their competence (Dunn *et al.* 2000; Storey 2001).

Remember!

Student effort is directly related to clinical competence. Using your portfolio is a way of demonstrating this effort.

Casey's (2001) pilot study on the assessment of clinical competence supported claims that the portfolio facilitates student development (Murrell *et al.* 1998; Griffin 2001; McMullan *et al.* 2003). Results of Casey's study demonstrate that a competency system that incorporates the use of a portfolio is viewed as a welcome alternative to the previously used approaches. Extending the uses of the portfolio, Murrell *et al.* (1998) declare that it facilitates the integration of theory with practice and allows students to assume ownership and control of their own learning needs. In contrast, although portfolios were well received by nursing students, Gallagher (2001) proposed the theory–practice link is not as strong as anticipated and could be associated with the students' 'limited autonomy' in the development of their portfolios. Nonetheless, the concepts of student ownership, responsibility and ongoing development associated with the use of the portfolio are central to adult education and motivation (Quinn 2000; Welsh and Swann 2002) and are therefore of particular significance to your development of competence as a student.

The significance of reflection for competence development may also be apparent through its association with the development of skills such as critical thinking skills (Nagayda *et al.* 2005). These skills are deemed an essential component and outcome of registration programmes that prepare students for professional nursing practice (Bell *et al.* 2002; Tzeng and Ketefian 2003) and are identified as fundamental to competent nursing practice (May *et al.* 1999). May *et al.* (1999) test the relationship between critical thinking skills and clinical competence. These authors report that competent practice seemed dependent on critical thinking abilities. However, May *et al.* reaffirm that the relationship between critical thinking and clinical competence remains unclear (Maynard 1996). Bell *et al.* (2002) note paucity within the literature that investigated how to promote undergraduate nursing students' critical thinking abilities.

Remember!

Use of reflection within your portfolio may develop your critical thinking skills.

There are few descriptions of the exact nature of competence assessment using portfolios for undergraduate nursing students, so providing practical examples is thus limited. The use of the portfolio to assess clinical competence in a postgraduate nursing situation in the Republic of Ireland is described in the literature (Coffey 2005). This author suggests 'the assessment of clinical competence in post-registration programmes requires redefinition of focus and techniques to capture the context of specialist practice'. Furthermore, it is suggested that the portfolio is preferred as a method of providing 'snapshots of clinical learning' that can be 'assembled and combined to reveal a more holistic impression of the learning experience' (Coffey 2005). In this way, you as a student can compile your snapshot of clinical learning, and include it in portfolio presentation. This is one example of the more holistic view that can be taken with portfolio use. Coffey (2005) describes the use of a portfolio to assess clinical learning and competence among a group of students attending a Higher Diploma in Gerontological Nursing. The author chose the portfolio as a measure of competence as it provided for the nurses' own initiative and experience and encouraged reflection and critical thinking. The full assessment (the portfolio) comprised three separate component parts: a portfolio of 'evidence-based practice development', 'an exemplar of reflection on practice' using a model of reflection (Johns 1995) and a record of clinical learning.

Good practice model for the use of the portfolio as an assessment tool

The full assessment (the portfolio) included:

- a portfolio of 'evidence-based practice development';
- 'an exemplar of reflection on practice' using a model of reflection (Johns 1995);
- A record of clinical learning.

(Coffey 2005)

A framework derived from core concepts of the role of clinical nurse specialist (NCNM 2003) was used to provide structure to the portfolio overall (Coffey 2005) (Table 4.1). This incorporates items that are identified as core elements of specialist practice. These are clinical focus, patient advocate, education and training, audit and research and consultant. An approach using these same core competencies was also used for postgraduate portfolio competence assessment by Joyce (2005). Students initially undertaking the portfolio found it a daunting experience, but their overall views were mostly positive (Coffey 2005). Support of local managers was deemed vital to the operation of the process.

Table 4.1 Core concepts of the role of clinical nurse or midwife specialist (CNS/CMS)

1. *Clinical focus*: The role of CNS must have strong patient focus whereby the specialty defines itself as nursing (or midwifery) and subscribes to the overall purpose, functions and ethical standards of nursing. The clinical practice role may be divided into two categories, direct and indirect care. Direct care comprises the assessment, planning, delivery and evaluation of care to patients and their families; indirect care relates to activities that influence others in the delivery of direct care.

2. *Patient advocate*: The CNS/CMS role involves communication, negotiation and representation of the client/patient values and decisions in collaboration with other professionals and community resource providers.

3. *Education and training*: The CNS/CMS remit for education and training consists of structured and impromptu educational opportunities to facilitate staff development and patient education. Each CNS is responsible for his/her own continuing education through formal and informal educational opportunities thus ensuring continued clinical credibility amongst nursing, medical and paramedical colleagues.

4. *Audit and research*: Audit of current practice and evaluation of improvements in the quality of patient care are essential. The CNS/CMS must keep up to date with current relevant research to ensure evidence-based practice and research utilization. The CNS/CMS must contribute to nursing research, which is relevant to his/her particular area of practice.

5. *Consultant*: Inter and intra-disciplinary consultations both internal and external are recognized as key functions of the clinical nurse/midwife specialist; this consultative role also contributes to improved patient client management.

Source: Coffey (2005) (with permission of Blackwell Science).

Most students agreed that the portfolio served as an effective measure of competence (Coffey 2005).

Much of the literature addressing the development of competence within the student nurse supports the use of portfolios to foster the development of reflective and critical thinking skills for competence development and professional practice. However, it remains unclear within the research how these concepts interact to achieve competence (Maynard 1996; May *et al.* 1999; Gallagher 2001), or indeed how practically the competence assessment interacts with the portfolio document. In some cases the portfolio is used to support a particular judgement of competence, perhaps from observation, and in others the portfolio itself provides the sole evidence of competence in a particular aspect of nursing. There are also situations where students develop a portfolio, but it has little or no formal link to the assessment of competence other than a casual observation by a registered nurse.

Remember!

Much of the literature addressing the development of nursing student competence supports the use of portfolios to foster development of reflective and critical thinking skills for competence development and professional practice.

However, despite the positive findings that exist in relation to the portfolio as a component of a holistic approach to competence assessment, some issues arise that warrant some discussion. In a paper exploring the use of portfolios in nurse education, Gannon and colleagues (2001) draw attention to a number of problems associated with the credibility of the portfolio as a learning tool and, more crucially, in the assessment of competence. They highlight a lack of consistency in theoretical underpinning and purpose, raise questions about honesty and confidentiality, and call into question the validity and reliability of portfolios as assessment tools. Their point in relation to the theoretical underpinning is a good one: although we now understand some of the origins of the portfolio from preceding chapters, particularly in relation to self-directed learning as outlined in Chapter 1, the origins, aims and purpose are often not clear to all those involved. The issue in relation to honesty is a thorny one, and it is speculated, and sometimes reported, that students do not give honest accounts, particularly in relation to their reflections, in part through embarrassment about revealing their innermost feelings to a relative stranger. This in itself is a finding, and may suggest that the portfolio process requires more of the facilitation process that is alluded to in Chapter 1 and will be considered in more detail in subsequent chapters.

Some theorists have raised the questionable assumption that the quality of the students' written work in their portfolio could be viewed as a reflection of their performance in practice (Gerrish et al. 1997; Calman et al. 2002). Perhaps if one were to consider the portfolio as the sole form of evidence for clinical competence this could indeed be problematic, as you as a student could potentially exaggerate your ability. However, from the literature it appears that portfolio use is intended within the construct of holistic competence assessment and therefore would represent one element in a range of evidence that may be used to support competence. Remember that a portfolio is a means of containing, developing and maintaining an appropriate collection of evidence; contemporary definitions do not profess that the portfolio itself is a measure of competence. Interestingly, in Coffey's (2005) earlier example, the portfolio was used in a holistic way to assess the competence of registered nurses attending a higher diploma programme. However, the assessment also included a record of clinical practice, which if used for nursing students could embrace the more behaviourist approach to assessment, with staff signing when key skills have been observed. This one example demonstrates that competence assessment with portfolio use rarely relies on one method alone.

Remember!

A portfolio is a collection and cohesive account of work-based learning that contains relevant evidence from practice and critical reflection on this evidence.

> Its primary purpose is to display the achievement of professional learning outcomes and knowledge development. However, an inherent aim is the encouragement of personal development.

There is also some concern by academics about the potential for the portfolio to be viewed as, or rendered an academic exercise rather than a true reflection of the students' practice and development of competence (Gerrish *et al.* 1997; Calman *et al.* 2002). The extent to which this is possible or occurs is related to the initial planning and preparation for the portfolio. If the portfolio has clear guidelines for the student, and is used to support particular aspects of student competence in the practical domain, and if a mentor or preceptor is required to facilitate your learning as a student, then it is more likely to remain enmeshed in the practice environment in keeping with the ultimate intention. The prospect of a portfolio becoming an academic exercise is not a pathway that students favour either. The additional effort required, combined with completing a clinical placement, can be arduous, particularly if this is a formative assessment, so it is important that School staff create mechanisms to avoid this occurrence.

When a simple pass or fail is given to a portfolio as part of summative assessment, this can be misleading as it implies that competence may be construed as absolute, whereas a continuum of competence is more likely to exist (Webb *et al.* 2003). However, in some cases there has been resistance to grading clinical performance. It has been noted that educators in Australia also consider it inappropriate to grade assessment of student clinical practice performance (Andresen *et al.* 2000). However, Andresen *et al.* argue that by combining both criterion-referenced and norm-referenced assessment, graded assessment can help students to understand better what constitutes minimal levels of competency, and at the same time recognize and reward meritorious practice.

The role of the external examiner in scrutinizing portfolio assessment is clearly important. Like other written assessments it comprises physical evidence that can be reviewed at a time and in a place distant from its origins. However, as a number of commentators have pointed out, external review of clinical practice assessment that is inviting an external examiner to review these assessments is problematic for practical reasons (Gerrish *et al.* 1997; Armitage and Karagic 2004). This requires considerable time investment by the examiner, or the use of video recorded assessments, and is not usual practice. In reviewing the activities of external examiners in England, the English National Board concluded that their role in monitoring practice assessment was at best minimal and at worst non-existent (English National Board for Nursing 2001). They draw attention to a lack of parity with theoretical assessment and highlight factors that militate against the external examiner's engagement with practice staff and practice assessment. They point out that the role of the external examiner continues to be poorly understood, that the current system of recruitment is unsatisfactory, and that the system pays only lip service to placement learning. They call for a joint agreement between the regulatory body and higher education sector on the role of the external examiner, with particular regard to the observation and scrutiny of competence assessment.

With reference to qualified nurses, Hull *et al.* (2005) suggest that the whole purpose of a portfolio is to develop reflective skills. However, it is clear from this discussion that portfolio use within nurse education settings is far more pervasive. It is used in a variety of ways either to contribute to or form the mainstay of competence assessment. The measurement of competence itself is complex, surrounded by debate within the nursing literature and compounded by the use of a multiplicity of terms. It is important that where portfolios are used, particularly within the context of competence, staff strive to develop rigorous guidelines to support their development adequately. It is also important that valid and reliable systems of assessment are in place, that students are facilitated in practice and that both staff and students receive adequate education on the processes.

Conclusion

Much of the literature on this area originated in the UK and Australia. Many papers highlight the complexity and confusion surrounding the concept of competence and the way in which it is defined, operationalized and assessed. There is a plethora of anecdotal and descriptive literature addressing competence and the tools that assess competence. Although limitations to the reviewed literature are recognized, research supports the need for any approach used for the development of competence to be a valid and reliable approach that is both patient-centred and focused on caring and professional practice.

Research also advocates the need for competence development to be holistic in nature; this includes the use of portfolios to support the assessment of competence. It emerges from the literature that holistic competence approaches increase student effort, participation, control, motivation and development. These factors are said to be most conducive to adult learning and nurse education thereby enhancing the notion of student development through competence-based approaches. In keeping with the findings of the literature and the concept of adult leaning, the use of the portfolio to support competence assessment is encouraged and is positively viewed by students. However, it is acknowledged that considerably more research and development is required in the area of both competence assessment and portfolio use, particularly in relation to the potential development of nationally validated tools.

Summary of key points

- The measurement of clinical competence is a modern approach to the assessment of nursing students in practice.
- Sometimes both students and nurses can be unclear as to the exact meaning of competence.
- Portfolios are used to provide supporting evidence for competence assessment and allow for greater student involvement.

Recommended further reading

Watson, R. *et al.* (2002) Clinical competence assessment in nursing: a systematic review of the literature, *Journal of Advanced Nursing*, 39(5): 421–31.

References

Alinier, G. (2003) Nursing students' and lecturers' perspectives of objective structured clinical examination incorporating simulation, *Nurse Education Today*, 23: 419–26.

An Bord Altranais (2000) *The Code of Professional Conduct for Each Nurse and Midwife*. Dublin: An Bord Altranais.

Andresen, L., Boud, D. *et al.* (2000) Experience-based learning, in G. Foley (ed.) *Understanding Adult Education and Training*. Sydney: Allen & Unwin.

Armitage, H. and Karagic, L. (2004) 'In name only'. Quality in practice assessment – is there a place for the external examiner?, *Nurse Education in Practice*, 4: 1–2.

Ashworth, P. and Morrison, P. (1991) Problems of competence-based nurse education, *Nurse Education Today*, 11(4): 256–60.

Baramee, J. and Blegen, M. A. (2003) New graduate perception of clinical competence: testing a causal model, *International Journal of Nursing Studies*, 40: 389–99.

Bell, M. L., Heye, M. L. *et al.* (2002) Evaluation of a process-focused learning strategy to promote critical thinking, *Journal of Nursing Education*, 41: 175–7.

Benner, P. E. (1984) From Novice to Expert: Excellence and Power in Clinical Nursing Practice. Menlo Park, CA: Addison-Wesley.

Bradshaw, A. (1997) Defining' competency' in nursing (Part I): a policy review, *Journal of Clinical Nursing*, 6(5): 347–54.

Bradshaw, A. (1998) Defining'competency' in nursing (Part II): an analytical review, *Journal of Clinical Nursing*, 7(2): 103–11.

Calman, L., Watson, R. *et al.* (2002) Assessing practice of student nurses: methods, preparation of assessors and student views, *Journal of Advanced Nursing*, 38(5): 516–23.

Casey, B. (2001) *Pilot Project for the Assessment of Clinical Competence*. Dublin: Assessment of Competence Conference, An Bord Altranais.

Cattini, P. and Knowles, V. (1999) Core competencies for clinical nurse specialists: a usable framework, *Journal of Clinical Nursing*, 8: 505–11.

Chambers, M. A. (1998) Some issues in the assessment of clinical practice: a review of the literature, *Journal of Clinical Nursing*, 7(3): 201–8.

Chapman, H. (1999) Some important limitations of competency-based education with respect to nurse education: an Australian perspective, *Nurse Education Today*, 19(2): 129–35.

Coffey, A. (2005) The clinical learning portfolio: a practice development experience in gerontological nursing, *Journal of Clinical Nursing*, 14(2): 75–83.

DoH (1999) *Making a Difference*. London: Department of Health.

Dolan, G. (2003) Assessing student nurse clinical competency: will we ever get it right?, *Journal of Clinical Nursing*, 12(1): 132–41.

Duffy, K. (2004) *Failing Students: A Qualitative Study of Factors that Influence the Decisions Regarding the Assessment of Students' Competence to Practise*. London: Nursing and Midwifery Council.

Dunn, S., Lawson, D. *et al.* (2000) The development of competency standards for specialist critical care nurses, *Journal of Advanced Nursing*, 31(2): 339–46.

English National Board for Nursing (2001) *Placements in Focus*. London: English National Board for Nursing.

Eraut, M. (1998) Concepts of competence, *Journal of Interprofessional Care*, 12(2): 127–39.

Fitzpatrick, J. M., While, A. E. *et al.* (1996) Operationalisation of an observation instrument to explore nurse performance, *International Journal of Nursing Studies*, 33(4): 349–60.

Foster, T. and Hawkins, J. (2004) Performance of understanding: a new model for assessment, *Nurse Education Today*, 24: 333–6.

Gallagher, P. (2001) An evaluation of a standards-based portfolio [corrected and republished article originally printed in Nurse Education Today, 21(3): April 2001: 197–200].

Gannon, F. T., Draper, P. R. *et al.* (2001) Putting portfolios in their place, *Nurse Education Today*, 21(7): 534–40.

Garrett, B. M. and Jackson, C. (2006) A mobile clinical e-portfolio for nursing and medical students, using wireless personal digital assistants (PDAs), *Nurse Education in Practice*, 6(6): 339–46.

Gerrish, K., McManus, M. *et al.* (1997) *Levels of Achievement: A Review of the Assessment of Practice*. London: English National Board for Nursing, Midwifery and Health Visiting.

Girot, E. (1993) Assessment of competence in clinical practice – a review of the literature, *Nurse Education Today*, 13:(83–90).

Gonczi, A. (1999) Competency-based assessment in the professions in Australia, *Assessment in Education*, 1: 27–44.

Government of Republic of Ireland (1998) *Report of the Commission on Nursing: A Blueprint for the Future*. Dublin: The Stationery Office.

Griffin, C. (2001) *The Development of Competencies for Registration*. Dublin: Assessment of Competence Conference, An Bord Altranais.

Griffith, J. R., Warden, G. L. *et al.* (2002) A new approach to assessing skills needs of senior managers, *Journal of Health Administration Education*, 20(1): 75–98.

Hull, C., Redfern, J. *et al.* (2005) *Profiles and Portfolios: A Guide for Health and Social Care*. Basingstoke: Palgrave Macmillan.

Jasper, M. (2006) Portfolios and the use of evidence, in M. Jasper (ed.) *Professtional Development, Reflection and Decision Making*, pp 154–183 Oxford: Blackwell Publishing.

Johns, C. (1995) Framing learning through reflection within Carper's fundamental ways of knowing in nursing, *Journal of Advanced Nursing*, 22(2): 226–34.

Joyce, P. (2005) A framework for portfolio development in postgraduate nursing practice, *Journal of Clinical Nursing*, 14(4): 456–63.

Lenburg, C. B. (2000) Promoting competence through critical self-reflection and portfolio development: the inside evaluator and the outside context, *Terressee Nurse*, 63(3) 11, 14–15, 18, 20.

Lofmark, A. and Wikblad, K. (2001) Facilitating and obstructing factors for development of learning in clinical practice: a student perspective, *Journal of Advanced Nursing*, 34(1): 43–50.

McMullan, M., Endacott, R. *et al.* (2003) Portfolios and assessment of competence: a review of the literature, *Journal of Advanced Nursing*, 41(3): 283–94.

May, B. A., Edell, V. *et al.* (1999) Critical thinking and clinical competence: a study of their relationship in BSN Seniors, *Journal of Nursing Education*, 38: 100–10.

Maynard, C. (1996) Relationship of critical thinking ability to professional nursing competence, *Journal of Nursing Education*, 35(1): 12–18.

Miller, G. E. (1990) The assessment of clinical skills/competence/performance, *Academic Medicine*, 65(9): S63–S67.

Milligan, F. (1998) Defining and assessing competence: the distraction of outcomes and the importance of educational process, *Nurse Education Today*, 18(4): 273–80.

Murrell, K., Harris, L. *et al.* (1998) Using a portfolio to assess clinical practice, *Professional Nurse*, 13: 220–3.

Nagayda, J., Schindehette, S. *et al.* (2005) *The Professional Portfolio in Occupational Therapy Career Development and Continuing Competence*. Thorofare, NJ: Slack Incorporated.

NCNM (2003) *Agenda for the Future Development of Nursing and Midwifery*. Dublin: National Council for the Professional Development of Nursing and Midwifery.

Neary, M. (1999) Preparing assessors for continuous assessment, *Nursing Standard* 13(18): 41–7.

NMC (2004) *Standards of Proficiency for Pre-registration Nursing Education*. London: Nursing and Midwifery Council.

Priest, H. and Roberts, P. (1998) Assessing students' clinical performance, *Nursing Standard*, 12(48): 37–41.

Queensland Nursing Council (2001) *An Integrative Systematic Review of Indicators of Competence for Practice and Protocol for Validation of Indicators of Competence*. Brisbane: Queensland Nursing Council.

Quinn, F. M. (2000) *The Principles and Practice of Nurse Education*. Cheltenham: Nelson Thornes.

Ramritu, P. L. and Barnard, A. (2001) New nurse graduates' understanding of competence, *International Nursing Review*, 48: 47–57.

Robb, Y., Flaming, V. *et al.* (2002) Measurement of clinical performance of nurses: a literature review, *Nurse Education Today*, 22: 293–300.

Scholes, J., M. Freeman, et al. (2004) *Evaluation of Nurse Education Partnership: Final Report*. Brighton: Centre of Nursing and Midwifery Research University of Brighton.

Shanley, E. (2001) Misplaced confidence in a profession's ability to safeguard the public?, *Nurse Education Today*, 21: 136–42.

Sinclair, M. and Gardner, J. (1999) Planning for information technology key skills in nurse education, *Journal of Advanced Nursing*, 30(6): 1441–50.

Storey, L. (2001) *The Concept of Competence*. Proceedings of the Assessment of Competence, Conference, Killiney, Co. Dublin. Dublin: An Bord Altranais.

Storey, L. and Haigh, C. (2002) Portfolios in professional practice, *Nurse Education in Practice*, 2(1): 44–8.

Tzeng, H. M. and Ketefian, S. (2003) Demand for nursing competencies: an exploratory study, *Journal of Clinical Nursing*, 12: 509–18.

UKCC (1999) *Fitness for Practice*. London: United Kingdom Central Council for Nursing, Midwifery and Health Visiting.

Urdang, L. (ed.) (1992) *The Concise Oxford English Dictionary*. Oxford: Oxford University Press.

Watkins, M. J. (2000) Competency for nursing practice, *Journal of Clinical Nursing*, 9(3): 338–46.

Watson, R., Stimpson, A. *et al.* (2002) Clinical competence assessment in nursing: a systematic review of the literature, *Journal of Advanced Nursing*, 39(5): 421–31.

Webb, C., Endacott, R. *et al.* (2003) Evaluating portfolio assessment systems: what are the appropriate criteria?, *Nurse Education Today*, 23(8): 600–9.

Welsh, I. and Swann, C. (2002) *Partners In Learning: A Guide to Support and Assessment in Nurse Education*. Oxford: Radcliffe Medical Press.

While, A. E. (1994) Competence versus performance: which is the more important?, *Journal of Advanced Nursing*, 20(3): 525–31.

Wilson-Barnett, J., Butterworth, T. *et al.* (1995) Clinical support and the Project 2000 nursing student: factors influencing this process, *Journal of Advanced Nursing*, 21(6): 1152–8.

Worth-Butler, M. M., Fraser, D. M. *et al.* (1996) Eliciting the views of experienced midwives about the assessment of competence in midwifery, *Midwifery*, 12(182–90).

Zhang, Z., Luk, W. *et al.* (2001) Nursing competencies: personal characteristics contributing to effective nursing performance, *Journal of Advanced Nursing*, 33(4): 467–74.

5

Portfolio Content

Fiona Timmins

Introduction • Relevant material for inclusion in the portfolio • What should the portfolio look like? • Putting it all together • Conclusion • Summary of key points • Recommended further reading • References

Introduction

As discussed previously, many Schools of Nursing now use the portfolio as a method of both formative and summative assessment (Rassin *et al.* 2006). It is commonly used as a combination approach to the holistic assessment of competence. This later development is positively received by students and can increase student satisfaction through increased student ownership and effort. Preparing a portfolio can be a daunting experience initially for students, although ultimately students find great satisfaction and indeed pleasure in the process (Tiwari and Tang 2003). It can help to reduce the perception of a gap between classroom teaching and clinical learning (Dolan *et al.* 2004; Endacott *et al.* 2004). Students suggest that the portfolio helps them to gain a greater understanding of practice, to apply their learning to professional practice and to learn deeply and conceptualize at a high cognitive level (Tiwari and Tang 2003). Other benefits include freedom in learning and increased confidence (Tiwari and Tang 2003). Students also report that a portfolio can enhance their professional skills, although students did not view it as a high priority on their course (Corcoran and Nicholson 2004).

Student benefits from using portfolios

- Greater understanding of practice.
- Ability to apply learning to professional practice.
- Fostering of deep learning and ability to apply classroom learning to professional nursing practice and conceptualize at a high cognitive level.
- Increased satisfaction with learning.
- Increased ownership of learning.

(Tiwari and Tang 2003)

A portfolio is a collection and cohesive account of work-based learning that contains relevant evidence from practice and critical reflection on this evidence. Its primary purpose is to display achievement of individual or organizational learning goals and knowledge development. Portfolio use within nurse education generally has a focus on learning from nursing practice. While some portfolios are either completed within the classroom setting or as a set assignment, they usually comply with this broad premise. More commonly the portfolio is a handheld document, such as a ring binder, that students carry with them and develop while they are actually gaining their experience within the clinical practice environment. Portfolios are firmly entrenched in learning from practice (Hull *et al.* 2005). However, there is an anomaly here in that very often the outcome of the portfolio is inherently personal to the individual student, as one of the main professed outcomes of portfolio use is personal development (Hull *et al.* 2005). The personal and private aspect of portfolios is well documented with regard to registered nurses (Brown 1992; Hull *et al.* 2005; NCNM 2006).

Activity 1

Whether or not you have used a portfolio, do you believe that it is something that you ought to share with others?

What would prevent you wanting to share the portfolio contents with other people?

Would you be tempted to modify the description of events as described in the previous chapter? If so, why?

Write down your responses before proceeding with the chapter.

The suggested private nature of portfolios has obvious merit for registered nurses maintaining their personal profile and record of achievement; for the nursing student who is attempting to outline learning in practice this may be less appropriate. First, the registered nurse who maintains a portfolio or profile may not be obliged to display it to any other person without consent, and if he or she is obliged to submit evidence from a portfolio, they may be able to take selecting parts. Therefore the registered nurse, who is accountable for his or her own practice, takes ownership and responsibility for the portfolio. Nursing students, on the other hand, submit their portfolios to the university or School, and in many situations, assessments automatically become the property of the educational establishment. Nursing students' portfolios are therefore relatively public documents that are viewed by mentors/facilitators and/ or staff within the Nursing School.

However, of more pressing concern than the issue of privacy is the fundamental question of what material to include within the portfolio. In order to provide the cohesive account suggested in Chapter 2 and incorporate evidence that is relevant, taking time to consider appropriate material for inclusion within the portfolio is called for, in addition to consideration of its final presentation.

Remember!

The nursing student portfolio is not usually a private document and is subject to viewing by others.

Relevant material for inclusion in the portfolio

In response to portfolio requirements for registration, particularly in the UK, a range of textbooks and articles feature the development of portfolios for registered nurses. No particular distinction is made in the literature between portfolios for registered nurses and those of nursing students – indeed, the registered nurse's portfolio of professional development is suggested to commence at the beginning of your programme, developing as you progress through it (Jasper 2006). There is an expectation that upon completion of the programme you will have an understanding and awareness of the need for professional development through portfolio use (NMC 2004). However, Jasper (2006) outlines some subtle differences between the two. The portfolio for the registered nurse serves to demonstrate professional competence and may be used as supportive evidence for registration purposes with a governing body (Jasper 2006). The student portfolio, on the other hand, is viewed quite differently. It is usually a programme requirement, during the course of study, often designed to demonstrate the achievement of developing competence or specific learning outcomes (Jasper 2006). It is often subjected to objective assessment using predesigned criteria.

These latter points have important relevance for the type of material that you will consider for inclusion. The contents of the nursing student portfolio will ultimately vary according to the particular guidelines of the course of study, or the specific purpose. So clearly the first phase of development of the portfolio is careful scrutiny of the requirements, learning outcomes and guidelines. The absence of clear guidelines makes the portfolio a more onerous task for you as a student, particularly in the absence of facilitation. In this latter case it is likely that the portfolio will begin to become unwieldy and lack particular focus. This lack of focus may be linked to the fundamental basis of the portfolio – self-direction. While this approach has been popular in nurse education for over twenty years, as outlined in Chapter 1, the term itself may lead to misinterpretation. As we discovered, not all students are actually ready to be fully self-directed. Often it is only the higher achievers that actually get to this point of independence; certainly in the earlier stages of a course, and very often, support and guidance is required. Rather than leaving the portfolio contents up to you as a student it is helpful if some clear and specific guidelines are put in place. Emden *et al.* (2003) cite lack of 'constructive guidance in building a portfolio' as a major barrier to development. It is often the case that even when guidelines do exist, these are deliberately broad and vague, in keeping with the premise of adult learning, and 'the majority of guidelines for constructing a portfolio do not seek to prescribe what should be included or how it should be presented' (Hull *et al.* 2005). This can be a problem for you as a student as you struggle to select material for inclusion.

Rather than providing specific guidelines at this point it may be useful to consider what you think you would place in your portfolio and then consider these items against those described in the literature as generally included within portfolios.

Activity 2

Pause for a moment and consider what items you may like to include in your portfolio. Write these ideas down and consider them further as we progress through the chapter.

It is easy to begin collecting for a portfolio without being clear about its purpose (Jasper 2006). A portfolio should always be kept with a purpose in mind, and all items that are included are linked to this purpose. With regard to nursing student portfolios, their purposes can vary and include: assessment; ongoing record of progress and achievements; to demonstrate development as a practitioner; self-directed log of activities; a guide for self-direction; a tool to document reflective learning or part component of a personal development plan (Jasper 2006). It can also contribute evidence for competence assessment as described in Chapter 4. While registered nurses often have a 'carte blanche' with regard to portfolio development, students are usually provided with some road markings in terms of learning outcomes or competence frameworks (Jasper 2006).

The purpose of a nursing student portfolio may vary and may include the following:

- Assessment.
- Ongoing record of progress and achievements.
- Demonstration of development as a practitioner.
- Self-directed log of activities.
- As a guide for self-direction.
- As a tool to document reflective learning.
- As a part component of a personal development plan.
- Evidence for competence assessment.

(Jasper 2006)

Evidence in the portfolio is crucial; this helps to demonstrate the claims that you are making (Jasper 2006). However, the evidence cannot stand alone; it must be linked clearly to the matter that it supports (Jasper 2006). In this way the evidence is woven in carefully so as to allow conclusions to be drawn. It is not suitable simply to include a set of lecture notes or handouts, or to photocopy articles from a journal without providing the meaning and relevance for the reader (Jasper 2006). Jasper summarizes the types of evidence as either primary or secondary. The student constructs primary evidences. These may take the form of reflections, consideration of achievement of

---

Evidence within the portfolio

Primary evidence, constructed by the student:

- Reflections.
- Consideration of achievement of learning outcomes.
- Commentaries on experiences.
- Written critical incident analysis.
- Notes on clinical supervision meetings.

Secondary evidence, drawn from outside of the particular individual and placed within the portfolio:

- Copies of patient information leaflets.
- Protocols, letters or testimonials. Copies of articles or other written work.
- Marking feedback sheets.

(Jasper 2006)

---

learning outcomes, commentaries on experiences, written critical incident analysis, notes on clinical supervision meetings. Secondary evidence is that which is drawn from outside of the particular individual and placed within the portfolio, such as copies of patient information leaflets, protocols, letters or testimonials, copies of articles or other written work and marking feedback sheets (Jasper 2006).

Remember!

Evidence in the portfolio is crucial; this helps to demonstrate the claims that you are making.

Remember!

It is not suitable simply to include a set of lecture notes or handouts, or to photocopy articles from a journal without providing the meaning and relevance for the reader.

Letters or testimonials are less commonly included in nursing student portfolios although they are commonly suggested for the portfolio of a registered nurse (Hull *et al.* 2005) or other practitioners (Nagayda *et al.* 2005). Other items collated by registered practitioners include quotes that reflect values/beliefs; transcripts; awards/diplomas; evidence of conference attendance; samples of documentation and 'Thank you' letters from clients (Nagayda *et al.* 2005). This may be further subdivided into eight categories for presentation (Nagayda *et al.* 2005) (Box 5.1).

Box 5.1   Categories for presentation within a professional portfolio

1   Values, missions, goals.
2   Education.
3   Professional development.
4   Professional skills.
5   Professional presentation.
6   Service.
7   Expressions of support.
8   Personal.

Source: Nagayda *et al.* (2005).

Similarly, Hull *et al.* (2005) suggest nurses should outline personal information; general education; professional education; employment and continuing

---

Box 5.2 Potential subdivisions within a professional portfolio

Introduction (who am I, my experience and goals).
Introduction to my skills, knowledge and abilities.
Competencies, skills and knowledge – communication skills, skills in critical reflection, ability to work on own initiative.
Indirect evidence – testimonials.
Appendices.

Source: Hull *et al.* (2005).

---

professional development. A sample framework is suggested to guide potential subdivisions within a professional portfolio (Box 5.2). Some authors suggest thinking of your portfolio as a creative work of art, with several items included to build up this picture of one's life's work (Hull *et al.* 2005). Brown (1992) suggests including a wide range of evidence (Box 5.3). Similarly, Brooks *et al.* (1998) outline suggestions for structuring a portfolio for professional registered nurses. This includes job description; academic transcripts; clinical validations (such as audit); health records; management accomplishments; hospital work; writing skills (published articles); presentations; research grants and projects; compliments.

Box 5.3 Range of evidence suggested for inclusion in the portfolio

Evidence of learning from prior experience.
Testimonials.
Diaries.
Evidence of qualifications and registration with professional bodies.
Completed assignments.
Judgements, assessments, evaluations by others.
Reports on voluntary work.
Video/DVD recordings.
Leaflets, information, references.
Critical incidents.
Published material.
Core competencies.
Curriculum Vitae.
Photographs.

Source: Brown (1992).

This listing and collecting of artefacts is referred to as the 'file cabinet' approach (Nagayda *et al.* 2005), or merely an up-to-date record of achievements (Hull *et al.* 2005) with no necessity for cohesion between elements. The evidence stands alone. This is similar to the biographical portfolio described by Cooper (1999), which simply lists personal characteristics and achievements. This is rarely used by nursing students. The primary purposes of the file cabinet portfolio are storage and showcasing talents, abilities and experience (Nagayda *et al.* 2005). This description of the use of portfolios for professionals leads to confusion, as in general these nurses are collecting a range of evidence for the regulatory body, to demonstrate personal and professional development. Clearly this showcase approach to portfolio development, which is a common approach, is not entirely suitable for the undergraduate nursing student who is expected to provide a rationale for inclusion of items with clear explanations: 'Do not just throw things in without explaining why they are there' (Pearce 2003: 61). Pearce suggests that if subsections are used, they should be clearly marked. These can also be referred to in a title page and introduction. Relevance and comprehensiveness of evidence included are important and relate to quality. They expand the breadth and depth of the portfolio. Pearce (2003) suggests a contents page, a title page and an introduction to explain how the portfolio is organized, clarify what personal and professional developments are being discussed and outline what evidence is proposed to support these. Specified learning outcomes should be addressed. Overall the portfolio should be informative and authentic (Pearce 2003).

Activity 3

Reconsider the items for inclusion that you identified in Activity 2. How do these compare to those that have been suggested so far?

Can you think of a way of neatly organizing your work within a portfolio, or subdividing it?

There is no set template for inclusive content for nursing student portfolios. Wenzel *et al.* (1998) suggest the inclusion of course work, case studies, essays, letters of recommendation, accounts of life experiences, and evidence from a multitude of diverse learning sources demonstrating the desired outcome objectives Dolan *et al.* (2004) suggest that the portfolio may be divided into four sections: academic, planning and preparation; miscellaneous and career sections (Table 5.1). The latter section indicates that this portfolio is aimed at preparing final year students for their careers and ultimately preparing their future portfolios for PREP.

Rassin *et al.* suggest that one of the core components of educational portfolios should be a reflective student record of experiences, which would include analysis and synthesis of learning from these situations as well as explanation of changes to opinions or behaviours as a result of reflection (Rassin *et al.* 2006). The educational portfolio may also include opinions of colleagues or grades (Rassin *et al.* 2006).

Table 5.1 Suggested sections of the student portfolio

Section of the portfolio
Academic sections
1   Summative assessment (essays)
2   Essay planning and writing
3   Placements record
4   Record of academic progress
5   Referencing guidelines
6   Formative assessment (critical incidents)

Planning and preparation
7   Record of absences
8   Exam planning and techniques
9   Approaches to study

Miscellaneous
10   Summary of meetings
11   Life experiences
12   Expectations of nursing course

Career sections
13   Stress management
14   Career planning
15   CV
16   Self and group advocacy
17   Educational opportunities (PREP)
18   Factors affecting career choices
19   Job searching

Source: Dolan *et al.* (2004).

One issue with portfolio use for nursing students is its sometimes isolated and personalized use. The student portfolio is technically rooted in practice; it should promote learning in practice and perhaps not be considered in such isolation. Academics in Chapter 4 urged caution against allowing the portfolio to become an academic exercise, rather than a tool for developing practice-based learning outcomes. If the student portfolio does not engage in some way with the clinical area, there is a greater risk of this happening. However, more importantly, we may be teaching you as students to learn about practice in a very insular way. Nursing theorists, for example, consider the nursing situation in a holistic way, taking into account the nature of health, the environment, the nurse and the client. Both nurses and nursing students are encouraged to practise holistic nursing care. This, then, leads one to question why has the portfolio developed in some areas as a personalized insular document. Perhaps assessment has muddied the water here, leading the portfolio to become another student assignment and therefore ultimately personal.

While the individualistic approach to the portfolio is not necessarily wrong, the meaning and value of this learning can be called into question. This is particularly so when nurse educators question the merit of the portfolio, when students themselves attach little importance to it, and when the portfolio becomes a mere collection of artefacts with little or no cohesion. With issues of reliability and validity hanging over the whole process, and certainly assessment criteria can go some way towards addressing this, one way to address the validity of what is primarily knowledge development and scholarship is to embed the development of the portfolio firmly in practice, facilitated by a registered nurse. Another important element is the need for a cohesive approach or overarching framework to tie the parts of the portfolio together. This can be the learning outcomes from the course or module, personalized learning outcomes/needs or competencies derived from practice. This overarching framework serves to hang the portfolio together. It is useful to break the portfolio down into component parts such as 'entries', individual discussions on areas of practice related to competencies or learning outcomes. Care should be taken, however, when the portfolio is broken down by subsections in this way, that a dialogue is maintained throughout sections (Pearce 2003; Endacott *et al.* 2004).

Endacott *et al.* (2004) reveal that nursing students use four broad approaches to compiling portfolios, termed 'the shopping trolley', 'toast rack, 'the spinal column' and the 'cake mix'. When the shopping trolley (Figure 5.1) approach is taken, this literally means that portfolios are a collection of evidence such as lecture notes, articles, assignment feedback, which have little or no link to learning outcomes or competencies (Endacott *et al.* 2004). The student usually chooses inclusion material with little or no input from the mentor/facilitator, nurse or lecturer. This type of portfolio was least common at the research sites.

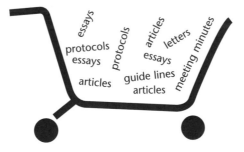

Figure 5.1 The shopping trolley approach to student portfolios

Source: Endacott *et al.* (2004). Copyright Elsevier.

A further category for the portfolios identified was the toast rack (Figure 5.2). This involved a portfolio made up of discrete elements separated within a ring binder, with little or no connection between parts. The authors noted an absence of an 'overarching narrative'.

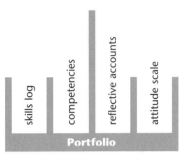

Figure 5.2 The toast rack approach to student portfolios

Source: Endacott *et al.* (2004).

A further conceptual model was the spinal column (Figure 5.3). The portfolio in this case is usually structured around competencies or learning outcomes, with evidence interspersed between. There is an emphasis on student originality here and the research team viewed this approach as more sophisticated than the approaches discussed above.

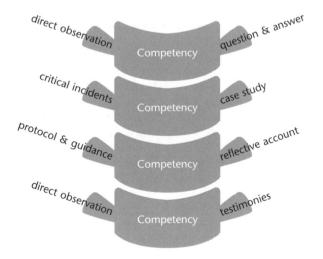
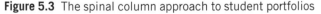

Figure 5.3 The spinal column approach to student portfolios

Source: Endacott *et al.* (2004). Copyright Elsevier.

The final approach noted, the cake mix (Figure 5.4), represents a full integration of both theory and practice. In this case there is evidence of an overarching narrative, like a reflective commentary. The portfolio becomes a whole rather than a series of parts. Reflexivity and development of practice were evident. This approach was guided by particular guidelines within the School of Nursing rather than independently provided by students.

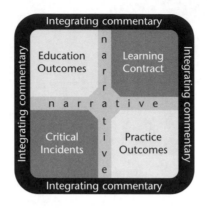

Figure 5.4 The cake mix approach to student portfolios

Source: Endacott *et al.* (2004). Copyright Elsevier.

The authors note that portfolio development appears developmental and evolutionary and that portfolios became more sophisticated over time. They suggest that Schools ought to provide greater guidance about appropriate use of evidence; encourage the use of the same evidence for a number of learning outcomes; prescribe limits to portfolio size and emphasize quality rather than quantity. They also suggested 'more emphasis on the student's input, with the use of dialogue pages, rather than focusing purely on assessor commentary' (Endacott *et al.* 2004: 254). Several factors are identified that influence the effectiveness of portfolios. First, the use of a robust structure such as the cake mix or spinal column is ultimately less time-consuming and clearly demonstrates an integration of theory with practice, promotes a greater understanding of practice and provides for a triangulation of evidence (see page 110). Appropriate guidance with realistic and consistent expectations of lecturers was also a contributory factor to success, including adequate preparation of staff and students.

Recommendations for Schools of Nursing using portfolios

- Provide greater guidance about appropriate use of evidence.
- Encourage the use of the same evidence for a number of learning outcomes.
- Prescribe limits to portfolio size.
- Emphasize quality rather than quantity.
- Encourage student input.
- Include student 'dialogue' pages, for student comment.
- Appropriate preparation for both staff and students.

(Endacott *et al.* 2004)

What should the portfolio look like?

It is possible to purchase ready-made portfolio frameworks that can provide the structure to a portfolio or profile (Hull *et al.* 2005); however, these may be more suited to registered nurses who are preparing these for their regulatory body. Several countries do provide either national (broad) guidelines, provide a framework at a low cost or recommend a privately purchased one.

One advantage with a purchased framework or one that is recommended to nurses within a particular country is consistency of use and application. This happens to be a particular weakness with portfolio use for nursing students. While at least some assessments within nurse education would have consistencies or similarities within specific areas, countries or indeed worldwide, the portfolio can sometimes be such a catch-all that anything goes. Although the contents and presentation vary, there has been little systematic review of the approaches used other than one recent UK study (Endacott *et al.* 2004). This study was particularly useful in demonstrating the variety of approaches taken by students within a single site, ranging from artefacts thrown together in a folder to a very cohesive, comprehensive, reflective account of learning from practice. These authors did suggest that portfolios are evolutionary and observed that as Schools of Nursing become more familiar with them and their drawbacks they begin to develop more stringent guidelines that improve overall quality. It could be said that there is confusion or misinterpretation of the purpose of portfolios. However, the accepted definitions, while straightforward, referring to a collection of evidence and reflection that attests to learning, usually from practice, may be misleading. Thus adding the term 'cohesive collection' prevents the mistaken assumption, as in the shopping trolley approach, that anything goes.

Remember!

A portfolio is a collection and cohesive account of work-based learning that contains relevant evidence from practice and critical reflection on this evidence. Its primary purpose is to display the achievement of individual or organizational learning goals and knowledge development. However, an inherent aim is the encouragement of personal development.

Very often the student portfolio is contained within a ring binder, which allows items to be removed and replaced (Dolan *et al.* 2004; Endacott *et al.* 2004; Hull *et al.* 2005), although electronic forms have been piloted with some success (Dagley and Berrington 2005). Certainly students express the desire to have something handheld and less bulky (Corcoran and Nicholson 2004). The use of a wireless personal digital assistant (PDA) as an electronic portfolio for students in Canada is described in the literature (Garrett and Jackson 2006). While the authors acknowledged that several paper-based portfolio initiatives were in existence, they developed a study to examine the potential benefit of electronic portfolios. Using a wireless mobile phone and digital camera-equipped PDA device to house the portfolio, the study aimed to identify students' views of this technology as a support to their learning in the clinical area and five themes emerged from the study including electronic reference v. interactive communication, interface limitations and reflection on practice. The students viewed the resources as a reference point rather than interactive material and found some of the resources provided very useful. The small screen deterred students from entries, as this was very time-consuming. They also found reflection while actually in practice difficult (Garrett and Jackson 2006). Although the authors were very positive about the device, few overall benefits in terms of portfolio development emerged.

Activity 4

Consider for a moment whether you prefer the notion of a ring binder portfolio or an electronic hand-held device?

Outline three advantages of both.

Outline three disadvantages of both.

Helpful tips regarding presentation are available from the literature on portfolios for registered nurses. The portfolio should be reader-friendly; ideally pages ought to be numbered or sequenced in some way; cross-referencing may be used to avoid repetition; appendices may be used for supporting information; clear headings and subheadings should be used; spelling and grammar should be checked and accurate and the layout should be consistent (NCNM 2006). Strong dividers may be used to differentiate clearly between sections (Hull *et al.* 2005). A glossary of terms can be helpful as well as a bibliography (Hull *et al.* 2005). Ultimately there should be evidence of scholarship and connections between sub-elements within (Hull *et al.* 2005). The portfolio approach should be selective, clear and concise, coherent and well presented. Connection between parts is important, to avoid either the shopping trolley or toast rack approach. This can simply mean providing a 'literature summary related to the student's perceived knowledge deficit in a specified area' (Levett-Jones 2007: 114) or incorporating simple dialogue between elements. Hayes *et al.* (2002) suggest the use of narrative as evidence to support the description of experiences or entries within the portfolio.

Remember!

- The portfolio should be reader-friendly.
- Pages ought to be numbered or sequenced in some way.
- Cross-referencing should be used to avoid repetition.
- Use appendices if you have a lot of supporting information.
- Use clear headings and subheadings.
- Check your spelling and grammar.
- Layout should be consistent.
- Strong dividers should be used to differentiate clearly between sections.
- Glossary of terms and a bibliography can be helpful.
- Provide evidence of scholarship and connections between sub-elements within.
- Ensure that evidence and contents are selective, clear and concise, coherent and well presented.
- Ensure connection between parts to avoid either the shopping trolley or toast rack approach.

Putting it all together

Emden *et al.* (2003) suggest a six-step portfolio building process for undergraduate students (Box 5.4). The inclusion of relevant evidence is often a source of confusion (Jasper and Fulton 2005).

Box 5.4   A six-step portfolio building process for undergraduate students

Choose skill areas (domains).
Agree learning outcomes (competencies).
Identify learning strategies (cues).
Identify performance indicators.
Collect evidence.
Organize evidence within the portfolio.

Source: Emden *et al.* (2003).

It is suggested that completeness of evidence rather than convergence is more important. Some portfolio models such as the shopping trolley and toast rack contain vast quantities of paper submitted as evidence, such as photocopied articles and lecture notes (Endacott *et al.* 2004). Pearce (2003) draws attention to the need to support each portfolio entry with evidence and to draw this evidence together with appropriate integration of theory, experience and research. She suggests a 'triangulation of evidence' (Pearce 2003: 33, fig 5.5). This involves reflecting on experience/s; then drawing on previous experience to interpret this; followed by considering the theory that exists or education received that may inform this observation; and finally supporting the reflection with evidence-based literature or evidence-based practice tools.

Jasper (1995: 449) outlines a workbook portfolio for nursing students that contributes to both formative and summative assessment: 'Used formatively the workbook enables the learning needs of the students to be identified, the acquisition of learning objectives monitored and the progress of the student continuously assessed'. The portfolio also forms part of a summative assessment with an examination. During the last six weeks of the programme the

Triangulation model

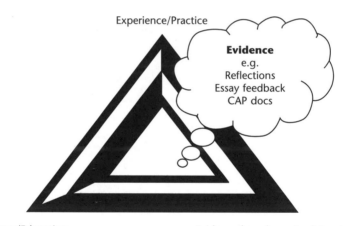

- Reflect on an experience, e.g. from practice.
- Draw on previous experience.
- Consider the theory that has informed the experience or practice, e.g. study day or theory learned at university.
- Support this with current literature or evidence-based practice tools.

By providing this triangulation of evidence you really demonstrate consideration of a wide range of resources, and it links all the essential qualities of professional practice.

Figure 5.5 Pearce triangulation of evidence

Source: Pearce (2003: 33).

student builds a 'model' client profile in the portfolio by relating themes to an actual client. Students are asked to: study in detail at least one aspect of care in relation to one patient; write a research-based nursing care plan; critique and evaluate the care received and reflect on their own actions and contributions with the 'aim of identifying knowledge and skill deficits and planning to remedy these' (Jasper 1995: 449).

Difficulty can occur with such a wide range of diverse, inclusive contents without specific direction, particularly for undergraduate nursing students who sometimes report confusion. In Chapter 1 of this book, a framework for construction of the portfolio emerges related to needs assessment for adult learners (Table 1.2).

Assessment of needs may relate to the specific programme requirements for the module or the experience, or needs related to competency. In order to achieve these needs, objectives are formulated and learning experiences are designed and planned. This may be simply stated as the range of experiences related to a particular clinical placement over a period of days or weeks, or these could be set experiences such as the decision to review an aspect of care or prepare a care study. The learning experiences may be subdivided in the folder according to domains of competence or standard of proficiency, or simply labelled as 'entries'. Within each of these entries a reflective account of experience/s can be included. There may also be references to textbooks or theory or evidence-based literature or evidence-based practice tools. All the time the framework for knowledge development (Figure 1.1) is kept in mind when developing the overarching theme that flows through the portfolio. So items need to be included and discussed that relate to this.

Remember!

Your learning experiences may be subdivided in the folder according to domains of competence or standard of proficiency, or simply labelled as 'entries'.

Conclusion

Students sometimes place little importance on the portfolio as a tool for personal development, skill development and information source, link between theory and practice or reflective tool (Dolan *et al.* 2004). It is also difficult for students to see the overall purpose and they report that they often receive too little input into portfolio preparation (Dolan *et al.* 2004). In particular they find the placing of evidence within the portfolio confusing (Corcoran and Nicholson 2004). On the other hand some see the benefits of the portfolio for their future professional development as registered nurses (Dolan *et al.* 2004). Some authors conclude that additional support is required (Corcoran and Nicholson 2004). Interestingly, many students do not perceive any difference in their delivery of care following completion of the portfolio (Corcoran and Nicholson 2004). Nevertheless, students do view the portfolio as an appropriate form of assessment that is fair and in fact easier to complete than some other assessments (Gallagher 2001). Some students report that it contributed positively to their learning and it was used as a learning resource for them (Gallagher 2001). Students also react favourably to the receipt of a grade for their work (Gallagher 2001), although negative views have also been reported (Mitchell 1994). Students may find it difficult to motivate themselves towards portfolios, but overall find that they encourage further reading (Mitchell 1994). Students perceive the use of structured models of reflection to be useful (Turner and Beddoes 2007). However, in the latter case the students did not receive a lecture on use of reflection and they found this a bit confusing. 'Developing a portfolio offers the opportunity for a student to identify and reflect on thoughts, theories explored, and decisions that resulted from particular work experience' (Hayes *et al.* 2002: 120). Resultant work can be very rich (Hayes *et al.* 2002). Key aspects to success within a portfolio are information, support, opportunity (reflective time) (Hayes *et al.* 2002).

Summary of key points

- Approaches to the structure of portfolios are varied.
- Professional portfolios for registered nurses may differ slightly in their approach.
- Endacott *et al.* (2004) reveal that nursing students use four broad approaches to compiling portfolios, termed 'the shopping trolley', 'toast rack, 'the spinal column' and the 'cake mix'.
- Students are encouraged towards a cohesive approach to the portfolio that relates component parts together using dialogue.

Recommended further reading

Endacott, R., Gray, M. A. *et al.* (2004) Using portfolios in the assessment of learning and competence: the impact of four models, *Nurse Education in Practice*, 4(4): 250–7.

References

Brooks, B., Barrett, S. *et al.* (1998) Beyond your resume: a nurse's professional 'portfolio', *Journal of Emergency Nursing*, 6: 555–7.

Brown, R. A. (1992) *Portfolio Development and Profiling for Nurses.* Lancaster: Quay.

Cooper, T. (1999) *Portfolio Assessment: A Guide for Lecturers, Teachers and Course Designers.* Perth: Praxis Education.

Corcoran, J. and Nicholson, C. (2004) Education Evaluation Research Learning portfolios – evidence of learning: an examination of students' perspectives, *Nursing in Critical Care*, 9(5): 230.

Dagley, V. and Berrington, B. (2005) Learning from an evaluation of an electronic portfolio to support general practitioners' personal development planning, appraisal and revalidation, *Education for Primary Care*, 16(5): 567–74.

Dolan, G., Fairbairn, G. *et al.* (2004) Is our student portfolio valued?, *Nurse Education Today*, 24(1): 4–13.

Emden, C., Hutt, D. *et al.* (2003) Exemplar. Portfolio learning/assessment in nursing and midwifery: an innovation in progress, *Contemporary Nurse*, 16(1–2): 124–32.

Endacott, R., Gray, M. A. *et al.* (2004) Using portfolios in the assessment of learning and competence: the impact of four models, *Nurse Education in Practice*, 4(4): 250–7.

Gallagher, P. (2001) An evaluation of a standards based portfolio [corrected and republished article originally printed in *Nurse Education Today*, 21(3), April 2001: 197–200].

Garrett, B. M. and Jackson, C. (2006) A mobile clinical e-portfolio for nursing and medical students, using wireless personal digital assistants (PDAs), *Nurse Education in Practice*, 6(6): 339–46.

Hayes, E., Chandler, G. *et al.* (2002) Nurse practitioner education. The master's portfolio: validating a career in advanced practice nursing, *Journal of the American Academy of Nurse Practitioners*, 14(3): 119–25.

Hull, C., Redfern, J. *et al.* (2005) *Profiles and Portfolios: A Guide for Health and Social Care.* Basingstoke: Palgrave Macmillan.

Jasper, M. (1995) The portfolio workbook as a strategy for student-centred learning, *Nurse Education Today*, 15(6): 446–51.

Jasper, M. (2006) Portfolios and the use of evidence in M. Jasper (ed.) *Professional Development, Reflection and Decision Making*, pp 154–183, Oxford: Blackwell Publishing.

Jasper, M. A. and Fulton, J. (2005) Marking criteria for assessing practice-based portfolios at masters' level, *Nurse Education Today*, 25(5): 377–89.

Levett-Jones, T. L. (2007) Facilitating reflective practice and self-assessment of competence through the use of narratives, *Nurse Education in Practice*, 7(2): 112–19.

Mitchell, M. (1994) The views of students and teachers on the use of portfolios as a learning and assessment tool in midwifery education, *Nurse Education Today*, 14(1): 38–43.

Nagayda, J., Schindehette, S. *et al.* (2005) *The Professional Portfolio in Occupational Therapy Career Development and Continuing Competence.* Thorofare, NJ: Slack Incorporated.

NCNM (2006) *Guidelines for Portfolio Development for Nurses and Midwives.* Dublin: National Council for Nursing and Midwifery.

NMC (2004) *Standards of Proficiency for Pre-registration Nursing Education.* London: Nursing and Midwifery Council.

Pearce, R. (2003) *Profiles and Portfolios of Evidence*. Cheltenham: Nelson Thornes.

Rassin, M., Silner, D. *et al.* (2006) Departmental portfolio in nursing – an advanced instrument, *Nurse Education in Practice*, 6(1): 55–60.

Tiwari, A. and Tang, C. (2003) From process to outcome: the effect of portfolio assessment on student learning, *Nurse Education Today*, 23(4): 269–77.

Turner, D. S. and L. Beddoes (2007) Using reflective models to enhance learning: experiences of staff and students *Nurse Education in Practice*, 7(3): 135–40.

Wenzel, L. S., Briggs, K. L. *et al.* (1998) Portfolio: authentic assessment in the age of the curriculum revolution, *Journal of Nursing Education*, 37(5): 209–12.

6

Portfolio Structure

Fiona Timmins

Introduction • Getting started • Using evidence within the portfolio
• Selecting a model of reflection • Conclusion • Summary of key points
• References

Introduction

A portfolio is a collection and cohesive account of work-based learning
that contains relevant evidence from practice and critical reflection on this
evidence. Its primary purpose is to display achievement of learning and
knowledge development. Portfolios may be used within education for both
summative and formative purposes. Summative portfolios focus on learning
outcomes and contain evidence that these are achieved. They aim to measure
students' skills or knowledge, and a grade or mark is awarded. Where the main
role of a portfolio is to demonstrate or encourage the learning process, but
where no final mark/grade is awarded, this is known as formative assessment.
It is likely that the type of summative portfolio that you are presented with
takes one of two common forms: either a competency-based portfolio, used in
conjunction with the curriculum to provide for appropriate assessment of clinical performance (Cooper 1999), or a negotiated learning portfolio, which
involves negotiating specific learning outcomes (Box 2.1).

Remember!

Portfolios that you are expected to complete as a component of a nursing programme may be awarded a mark/grade (summative assessment) or not (formative assessment).

The portfolio provides a method of developing students' reflective abilities and competence development (McMullan *et al.* 2003) and is sometimes designed solely to measure competence (Jasper 2006a). A formative portfolio may take several forms but would overall involve negotiating specific learning outcomes that are formatively rather than summatively assessed. Portfolios are most commonly used to provide supporting evidence for the competence assessment. However, approaches to competence measurement vary both nationally and internationally with resultant variety in the nature and presentation of linked portfolios.

As discussed in Chapter 4, competence may be conceptualized as comprising three main approaches: behaviourist, generic or holistic. You are reminded of these approaches and definitions below. Within nurse education, in the context of student-centred learning and adult approaches to learning, there is an impetus towards holistic models of competence development that incorporate the use of additional forms of evidence other than direct observation – hence the popularity of the portfolio. Student participation in and responsibility towards competence assessment are enhanced where portfolios are used in this holistic approach (Murrell *et al.* 1998; Griffin 2001; McMullan *et al.* 2003). The key to this success is thought to be the student's active engagement in the process (Murrell *et al.* 1998; Griffin 2001; McMullan *et al.* 2003).

Competency definitions combine three main categories:

- What students should be like.
- Attributes students need to possess.
- What students need to achieve.

Approaches to competence are further described:

- Behaviourist: necessitating the performance of a specified behaviour or task that can be observed or measured.
- Generic: referring to a cluster of generalized abilities.
- Holistic: including a mix of approaches such as cognitive, psychomotor and affective.

Remember!

Your active engagement in the process can improve the experience.

Whether or not competence measurement forms part of the portfolio, guidelines can vary and, in keeping with the momentum of the self-direction movement (Chapter 1), instructions can be vague or variable in terms of presentation, size and indeed content. Little precise direction emerges from an extrapolation of the literature on the topic in Chapter 5 that could assist you directly as a student to know exactly what to 'put in' the portfolio, or how to present it, other than some guiding principles. On the other hand, quite specific guidelines for portfolios used by qualified nurses feature quite heavily in the literature, and most suggest a biographical format. In this case the portfolio is mostly a collection vehicle for past achievements, in an extended Curriculum Vitae approach; however, this offers little by way of instruction to you as a student, as this approach is not usually suitable to your particular needs. With regard to general principles for the nursing student portfolio, there is general agreement that reflection forms a component of the portfolio and that the content should be linked together in a cohesive fashion. Broad presentation terms have been described according to Endacott *et al.* in Chapter 5 of this book as either: shopping trolley (Figure 5.1); toast rack (Figure 5.2), spinal column (Figure 5.3) or cake mix (Figure 5.4) depending on the integration of artefacts contained in the portfolio (Endacott *et al.* 2004), with an expressed preference for the two latter models. It is hoped that this chapter will provide further guidance on general portfolio structure.

General guiding principles of nursing student portfolio:

- Contains evidence of reflection.
- Gathers information together in a cohesive way.
- Presents information using a toast rack, spinal column or cake mix approach.

Getting started

Students often find it difficult to become motivated towards their portfolio. It has been reported that students sometimes fail to attach enough importance to the portfolio as a learning tool (Dolan *et al.* 2004). Students often find the portfolio confusing (Corcoran and Nicholson 2004) particularly if they are not versed in key inclusive features such as reflection (Turner and Beddoes 2007). However, you will be reassured that students who have used portfolios do report that it can contribute positively to their learning and be a useful learning resource (Gallagher 2001). In some surveys, students attach meaning and relevance to the portfolio and believe it to be a very appropriate mode of assessment (Harris *et al.* 2001). Nevertheless, while some students place value on the portfolio, their actual use of it can be very limited (Harris *et al.* 2001). In some cases students place a very low priority on the portfolio, and do not report using them frequently (Harris *et al.* 2001). The use of the portfolio for summative assessment and assigning a grade to the work appears to increase motivation towards completion, although this is also thought to inhibit students' creativity within the portfolio (Harris *et al.* 2001).

Activity 1

From your reading so far and your personal experiences, what are your views on the value of student portfolios?

Do you believe that achieving a grade or mark for a portfolio would increase your own motivation?

Write down your responses before you proceed with the chapter.

Attaching significance to the grading of portfolio work is interesting in this context, as it places significance on external motivation for learning when, contrarily, self-direction and independent motivation is the founding premise of portfolio use. The underpinning belief of the self-direction movement, as we found out in Chapter 1, is that adults are naturally motivated towards learning, without the necessity for external rewards. Are you more likely to be motivated by a grade? (Activity 1). With this in mind it must be remembered that there is an expectation that you will be able to motivate yourself and take responsibility for your learning, whether or not there is a grade awarded. As mentioned in Chapter 3, putting things off, or procrastination, is a human trait and commonly employed when portfolios need to be prepared! However, putting off an activity, as you know, can ultimately lead to last minute preparation and you may not achieve as much as you could from the process. Remember that the process, the 'doing', is just as important for your learning as the final product.

Remember!

The portfolio process, the 'doing', is just as important for your learning as the final product.

Don't put it off until the last minute.

It must be borne in mind that the premise here is that you are an adult learner, capable of independently identifying learning needs and goals and seeking out experiences to satisfy these. Although everyone will vary in the extent to which they can achieve this level of independence, most people ought to be capable of achieving some degree of self-direction. That is not to say of course that you do this completely alone. It is expected that you would obtain some supportive facilitation. This is an identified person with whom you can work through things to ensure that you are on the right track. This person will not necessarily direct you but rather work alongside you to encourage you to come up with your own solutions. Linking back to Chapter 1, and our discussion of adult learning, the first step is to establish what it is you are expected to do within the portfolio (a facilitator can help you to tease out your ideas here) and therefore establish your own personal needs (Table 1.2).

Remember!

It is expected that you would obtain some supportive facilitation. This is an identified person with whom you can work through things to ensure that you are on the right track. This person doesn't necessarily direct you but rather works alongside you to encourage you to develop solutions.

The next step is to establish whether there are clear guidelines for your portfolio, and seek clarification if required. Using the guidelines, or expected learning outcomes/activities, identify what it is you need to do to achieve the set goals. This will help you to assess your own specific learning needs. These can be simply written on a piece of rough work in the first instance and later transferred to the portfolio.

Activity 2

Think about your own personal learning needs related to the portfolio that you are about to prepare.

Write down some notes before you proceed with the chapter.

If your portfolio is linked to assessment of competence, as described in Chapter 4, then you may need to attend the clinical placement, complete practice/competence documentation, engage with practice under the guidance of a facilitator/mentor, participate in holistic client care and gain exposure to a range of health care situations. You may also have specific learning needs based on your own personal experience, and thus you may have individual needs. An example of this is 'I need to develop my communication skills'. Examples of these learning needs are provided in Box 6.1.

Box 6.1   Examples of identified learning needs within a
portfolio linked to competence assessment

Learning needs

I need to attend clinical placement for a specified period of time
_____.

I need to meet with my mentor/facilitator.
I need to complete practice/competence documentation by _____.
I need to engage with practice under the guidance of a facilitator/mentor.
I need to participate in holistic client care and gain exposure to a range of
health care situations.
I need to develop my communication skills.

Once the broad learning needs have been identified, these can be condensed
and used as the basis for formulating objectives. Objectives are specific outcomes related to the portfolio. Based on what it is that you are required to do,
and other additional needs that you have identified, what do you expect to
achieve from the portfolio?

Activity 3

What do I need to achieve from my portfolio?

Write down some notes.

Based on the needs identified above (Box 6.1), some possible objectives are
listed in Box 6.2.

If the portfolio is based upon negotiated learning outcomes (LO) then a
similar process takes place. Personal learning needs are identified based perhaps on personal areas of interest, areas in which knowledge may need to be
improved, or particular areas of relevance to the clinical area that you are
participating in.

From these latter notes your learning needs may emerge as follows: to gain
exposure to relevant experiences in the clinical area, to read research on

---

Activity 4

When your portfolio is not related to competence think about your own personal learning needs related to your areas of interest, any knowledge gaps or
areas that are of interest in the clinical area.

Write down some notes before you proceed with the chapter.

Box 6.2 Examples of portfolio objectives for portfolio linked to competence assessment

Portfolio objectives

To attain competence through full engagement and participation with the clinical practice environment.
To demonstrate learning within the domains of competence.
To ensure that competence documentation is completed accurately.
To further develop personal communication skills.

---

the topic and to reflect on experiences and reading (see example Box 6.3). Objectives may then be developed (see example Box 6.4).

In relation to presentation tips provided in the previous chapter (see reminders below), the outline of portfolio objectives may form the first insert

---

Box 6.3 Examples of portfolio objectives within a portfolio linked to competence assessment

Learning needs

I need to attend clinical placement for a specified period of time _____ .

I need to meet with my mentor/facilitator.
I need to gain exposure to relevant experiences in the clinical area.
Patient education, communication with patients _____
I need to read research on the topic and to reflect on experiences and reading.

Box 6.4 Examples of identified learning needs within a learning outcome-based portfolio

Portfolio objectives

To improve listening and attending skills.
To participate in or observe patient education sessions.
To read and analyse relevant research articles and theory related to objective 1 and 2.

---

into your portfolio ring binder with a plastic sleeve to allow easy removal and protection. The next task is to identify specific learning experiences. Where a portfolio is used to support competence assessment, the domains of competence or the competence framework are often used to subdivide the discussion and presentation of the learning experiences in a toast rack fashion (Figure 5.2). The portfolio aims to provide snapshots of clinical learning put together to reveal a holistic impression of the learning experience (Coffey 2005), so outlining learning experiences within each subsection will achieve this aim in terms of creativity, richness and variety.

For a reminder of what you should include in your portfolio, see the boxes on pages 99,101.

As previously discussed, the approaches to competence assessment internationally are multiple and varied. Although there are calls for nationally agreed competence frameworks, these have not yet been established (Calman *et al.* 2002). It is therefore not possible to outline here the variety of learning experiences that a particular approach to competence assessment may expect. However, quite simply, if the portfolio relates to competence assessment, the portfolio, and thus the learning experiences, may be subdivided according to categorization or subheadings employed by the competence assessment tools. Where portfolios are used as a holistic approach to competence assessment the use of an organizing framework to outline learning experiences, based in relevant domains of competence, have been successfully applied at postgraduate level (Joyce 2005).

Remember!

A portfolio is a collection and cohesive account of work-based learning that contains relevant evidence from practice and critical reflection on this evidence. Its primary purpose is to display the achievement of individual or organizational learning goals and knowledge development.

To summarize what we have learnt so far in relation to the preparation of your portfolio:

1 Identify your own personal learning needs; document these in the portfolio.
2 Establish whether there are clear guidelines for your portfolio, and seek clarification if required. Use the guidelines to format the portfolio.
3 Once your broad learning needs have been identified these can be condensed and used as the basis for formulating objectives. Objectives are specific outcomes related to the portfolio; document these in the portfolio.
4 Using the guidelines, or expected learning outcomes/activities, identify what it is you need to do to achieve the set goals. Use this to design or plan your learning experiences.

5 If your portfolio is linked to assessment of competence as described in Chapter 4, then you may need to attend the clinical placement, complete practice/competence documentation, engage with practice under the guidance of a facilitator/mentor, participate in holistic client care and gain exposure to a range of health care situations. You may also have specific personal learning needs based on your own previous experience.

6 Evaluate the process so far.

7 Select an approach to presentation (toast rack, spinal column or cake mix).

8 Select a model to underpin the overall approach.

Selecting one model to underpin the overall approach and construct the presentation of the portfolio that suits all purposes is inherently problematic. When the portfolio is used as an adjunct to competence assessment, tools and documents for the development and assessment of competence within the clinical area are underpinned by a wide variety of theoretical frameworks. Although there is a call for a more consistent approach nationally, as we discovered in Chapter 3, a plethora of competence assessment tools exist. If they are being used they will ultimately shape the portfolio approach. However, to explain how a competence-based approach may be utilized as a model to support the portfolio, some examples are provided. In the Republic of Ireland, for example, the regulatory body, An Bord Altranais, requires five domains of competence (Box 6.5) to be attained by each nursing student upon programme completion in order to satisfy entry to the professional register (An Bord Altranais 2004). Both the domains of competence and the performance indicators are clearly outlined in the document. These five domains form the basis of competence assessment across the country, and where these are in use the portfolio learning experiences could sensibly be categorized accordingly (An Bord Altranais 2004), in a toast rack fashion.

Box 6.5   Five domains of competence required for entry to the nursing register in the Republic of Ireland

1   Professional/ethical practice.
2   Holistic approaches to care and the integration of knowledge.
3   Interpersonal relationships.
4   Organizational and management of care.
5   Personal and professional development.

Source: An Bord Altranais (2004).

Activity 5

Consider one of these five domains of competence (Box 6.5).

Identify one to three potential learning needs that you may have in this area.

Identify learning objectives related to these needs.

Similarly in the UK, the National Nursing Council (NMC 2004) proffers four standards of proficiency for entry to the register that could be similarly used as a framework to outline learning experiences (Box 6.6). One potential drawback with the use of competence domains or standards of proficiency as a model of presentation is that this toast rack approach may discourage you as a student from connecting the subsections together. The temptation is to leave each piece of work within its neat section in its entirety, without considering its possible connection to the subsequent sections. While this approach has resulted in some very good examples of portfolio use, demonstration of cohesiveness is a requirement of the portfolio, and remains a challenge with this approach.

Activity 6

Consider one of these four standards of proficiency (Box 6.6)

Identify one to three potential learning needs that you may have in this area.

Identify learning objectives related to these needs.

Pearce (2003) further adapts one of these examples (NMC standards of proficiencies) (NMC 2004) and recommends them for particular for use within student portfolios, suggesting that the portfolio may be divided into the following subsections: developing professional and ethical practice; developing client care; developing management and clinical leadership and developing as a lifelong learner. The latter author suggests the proficiency standards as a recommended model for nursing student portfolios, regardless of whether the portfolio is linked to competence assessment or not. It is possible, therefore, even with personalized learning outcomes, that some or all of the relevant

---

Box 6.6   Four standards of proficiency required for entry to the UK Nursing Register National Nursing Council

1   Developing professional and ethical practice.
2   Care delivery.
3   Care management.
4   Personal and professional development.

Source: NMC (2004).

---

proficiency standards or domains of competence related to your specific area may be utilized to subdivide your description of your learning experiences.

Remember!

The portfolio may be divided into the following subsections regardless of the overall approach:

- Developing professional and ethical practice.
- Developing client care.
- Developing management and clinical leadership.
- Developing as a lifelong learner.

Alternatively, where the portfolio is based around negotiated learning outcomes (LO), these learning outcomes or portfolio objectives could also instead be used to subdivide or categorize within the portfolio. In the example above (Box 6.6) the related four subsections could be: listening and attending skills; patient education sessions; research and theory related to communication and patient education. While attempting to gain structure in what can become an unwieldy document, difficulties immediately emerge. With the suggestion of subdivision of the folder comes the risk that items will be placed in toast rack style without specific discussion, and one suggestion is that an overview of each item is provided (Karlowicz 2000). Furthermore, where competence assessment documents are used, where should the documents be placed? It is usually contained as one unit, although it may have inherent subsections. Perhaps the solution here is to place it in the appendix and refer to it within each discussion of the learning experiences within the domains of competence, or relevant subdivision within the portfolio. Learning experiences that are outlined then simply refer to the competence assessment document within the appendix.

Remember!

Where the portfolio is based around negotiated learning outcomes (LO) these learning outcomes or portfolio objectives could also instead be used to subdivide or categorize within the portfolio.

When subsections are used within the portfolio, regardless of what the headings relate to, there is a risk of disjointedness evidenced in the toast rack approach outlined in Figure 5.2 (Endacott *et al.* 2004). However, the approach overall provides for more cohesiveness than the shopping trolley model (Figure 5.1), where all artefacts are just placed in a folder with no specific connection emerging (Endacott *et al.* 2004). Ultimately the aim, in terms of presentation, is for either a spinal column or a cake mix approach (Figures 5.3 and 5.4) (Endacott *et al.* 2004). The use of a division according to domains of competence or portfolio objectives lends itself nicely to the spinal column approach (Endacott *et al.* 2004). It is important to remember that this delineation of your planned learning experiences into broad categories is not just a paper exercise, which can be a common criticism of the portfolio. It is meant to create 'resources and strategies to achieve the learning goal' (Knowles *et al.* 1998: 213). Various activities, such as those referred to in the spinal column approach (Endacott *et al.* 2004) outlined in Figure 5.3, will be employed to satisfy the learning need and the resultant evidence will be enclosed within. Examples of these are direct observation, outlining a patient case study, a reflective account, testimonies, use of protocols and guidelines. Evidence will be discussed in more detail later in the chapter. For now we are still examining ways to contain this learning tool and make it manageable so that meaningful learning may take place.

Adding some stages in portfolio building may enrich the emerging overarching framework in advance of overall evaluation of the learning experience, as suggested by Knowles (Knowles 1989; Knowles *et al.* 1998). These are identifying performance indicators and collection of evidence (Emden *et al.* 2003) (Box 6.7).

Within each domain of competence or proficiency standard, according to the approach being used locally, performance indicators should be readily available to you. These are more detailed descriptions of the type of knowledge, behaviours and skills required within each domain. Once identified, these guide the selection of evidence that will ultimately support the suggestion that you are competent in particular areas. It is important at this point to reiterate the need for the portfolio to be of manageable proportions. It may be difficult for nursing students, even as adult learners, to decide how much learning to include in the portfolio. It may be useful, as is common among portfolios used by teachers, to describe learning experiences within each category (domains/standards/learning outcome) as 'entries' that focus on one or two particular performance indicators. Each subsection may have more than one entry (this may be decided by the individual or the educational establishment) that each provides its own evidence. It is important to map your learning, somehow tying your learning together within each section (Price 2003). Box 6.8 displays one

---

Box 6.7 Suggested steps in building a portfolio

Assessment of needs (Knowles 1989).
Formulation of objectives (Knowles 1989).
The design of learning experiences (Knowles 1989).
Identifying performance indicators (Emden *et al.* 2003).
Collection of evidence (Emden, Hutt *et al.* 2003).
Evaluation.

Box 6.8   Example of proficiency standard and performance indicator

Proficiency standard	Developing professional and ethical practice.
Performance indicator	Demonstrates respect for patient and client confidentiality.

Source: NMC (2004).

---

national proficiency standard from the UK (NMC 2004) and a related outcome, which may be used as a performance indicator within the portfolio (Emden *et al.* 2003).

This performance indicator (Box 6.8) could be supported by an entry that comprises a summary of a research article and personal reflection, or by a colleague's testimony, or video of skill demonstration as evidence. Patients' contribution to competence assessment has been briefly suggested in the literature, although this is not a concept that has been developed further. It is likely that a patient testimony may also fit here if appropriate. In the case of multiple performance indicators, at some point you need to decide, perhaps in relation to personal learning needs, which of these you will select for specific entries within the portfolio. A minimum of two and maximum of six may be suggested. The evidence produced within each entry also needs to be carefully selected and clearly linked to the indicator, and not placed in an ad hoc fashion.

In relation to competence assessment, the assessment may ultimately be supported by a range of evidence, including the observations of the facilitator or mentor. The portfolio is not, therefore, usually required as an all-encompassing document defending competence, but rather as an adjunct support that provides a more holistic approach. This includes the acceptance of a range of evidence to support competence and student involvement. Learning outcome-based portfolios will similarly require the delineation of performance indicators that will be outlined to allow measurement of achievement of learning outcomes. Take the portfolio objective 1 in Box 6.4, 'to improve listening and attending skills'. A performance indicator for this objective may be 'demonstrates an understanding of the skill of listening and attending', or 'demonstrates skills of listening'. Once the performance indicators are outlined, the next step according to Emden (Emden *et al.* 2003) is the collection of evidence, the exact nature of which will now be considered.

Remember!

In relation to competence assessment, the assessment may ultimately be supported by a range of evidence, including the observations of the facilitator or mentor. The portfolio is not, therefore, usually required as an all-encompassing document defending competence, but rather as an adjunct support that provides a more holistic approach.

Using evidence within the portfolio

A further contribution to your use of a portfolio is the consideration of evidence. The use of evidence within a portfolio is crucial (Lyons 1998). Rather than this document spiralling into a personal manifesto based on anecdotes, each aspect of your portfolio should have some type of supporting evidence. Jasper (2003) highlights the importance of using evidence within your portfolio, as this enables you to support and validate your assertions (Jasper 2006a). Evidence is referred to as both primary and secondary (see box on page 99), and both are useful for this purpose.

Evidence within the portfolio for qualified nurses is varied and extensive and includes:

- biographical information;
- educational background;
- certification;
- employment history;
- résumé;
- competency record;
- personal and professional goals;
- professional development;
- presentations, consultations and publications;
- professional activities;
- community activities;
- honours and awards; and
- letters ('thank you' letters) (Williams 2003; Sherrod 2005).

For the nursing student the evidence must clearly link to the portfolio outcomes and link to the sub-headings, and performance indicators if used. Examples of evidence to be included are certificates of attendance at educational days, or reflective notes about this; notes and lists of a related programme of reading that you have done; observations from practice episodes, with a 'clear description' including how you felt and what you understood, and selected discussions with your mentor or preceptor (Price 2003). Structured reflection upon practice provides another form of evidence for your portfolio (Rassin et al. 2006).

Consider your communication with a patient during an assessment process, or while performing a nursing intervention. The educational portfolio may also include opinions of colleagues, testimonies or grades (Rassin *et al.* 2006), although this is a less common approach. Student evidence may also include assignments, competence documentation, attendance records, essay plans, approaches to study, summaries of meetings and exam planning techniques (Dolan *et al.* 2004). The list of relevant evidence appears endless, and you can easily see how this could get out of hand! It is also noted that the portfolio can be quite time-consuming for you as a student (Murray 1994) and may have no prescribed physical limit (word or size limit). Thus, in the absence of explicit recommendations about evidence to be included, there is again the risk, even in the presence of a domain/standards-based framework or learning outcome-based framework, of confusion and uncertainty.

Remember!

Common forms of evidence within portfolios include:

- A reflective student record of experiences.
- Analysis and synthesis of learning from these situations including explanation of changes to opinions or behaviours as a result of reflection (Rassin *et al.* 2006).
- Opinions of colleagues, testimonies or grades (Rassin *et al.* 2006).
- Assignments.
- Competence documentation.
- Attendance records.
- Essay plans.
- Approaches to study.
- Summaries of meetings.
- Exam planning techniques.

While it is often not made explicitly clear exactly what evidence should be contained within each portfolio, it is increasingly evident that the evidence should be relevant to the portfolio objectives and discussed in a meaningful way. This limits the inclusion of evidence to a certain extent. As previously mentioned, your portfolio can be divided into subsections related to particular performance indicators, each containing one or more entries. Using an example of a performance indicator, 'demonstrates an understanding of the skill of listening and attending', this could be supported by an entry that comprises the summary of a research article and personal reflection. Similarly, 'demonstrates skills of listening' may be a separate entry supported by a colleague's testimony or video of skill demonstration.

> **Remember!**
>
> While it is often not made explicitly clear exactly what evidence should be contained within each portfolio, it is increasingly evident that the evidence should be relevant to the portfolio objectives and discussed in a meaningful way.

> **Remember!**
>
> Each subsection may have several 'entries' supported by evidence.

As previously mentioned, you may need to provide a rationale for the number and choice of particular performance indicators. Evidence selected to support the indicator needs to be appropriate. The nature and type of evidence will vary according to the indicator being attained; however, in keeping with the aim of knowledge development, and from your reading in Chapter 1, it may be useful to consider evidence related to technical aspects of practice (such as descriptions of tasks performed, outline of patient conditions in text books, instructions for pharmaceutical preparations and technical equipment); rules, laws and regulations (practice guidelines, policies, procedures); tacit learning (your observations of practice) and a reflection on the latter forms of knowledge to gain a greater understanding of your personal tacit learning and social wisdom from practice, thus resulting in the combination of explicit and tacit knowledge, the collective and individual and thus the integration of the four forms of knowledge (Baumard 1999).

Although a distinct element outside the portfolio, reflection is a predominant theme in the literature in relation to portfolio use. Reflective accounts are frequently used as evidence within the portfolio. However, rather than simply thinking back on practice, a particular model of reflection is often suggested. However, the model of reflection needs to be reflected upon, thus we become more reflexive about our approach to the portfolio, and less likely to take current approaches for granted. The literature abounds with discussions regarding the use of models of reflection for both practice and education in nursing, and many challenges with their use emerge. As discussed in Chapter 3, there is a belief by some that the current use of reflection in nursing is overtly personal, and therefore questionable in terms of the nature of evidence it may provide. Reflection forms a component of most documented uses of portfolios within the literature and appropriate models of reflection in the context of knowledge development within the portfolio need further consideration. Furthermore, the model of reflection itself may form a cohesive approach or overarching framework to tie the parts of the portfolio together.

Reflection as an overarching framework serves to hang the portfolio together.

This will require some discussion and/or critical analysis of its contents, as is suggested, to provide the relevant evidence (Karlowicz 2000). Evidence of achievement of competence may be relevant evidence in this context. Another item that is often omitted from current student portfolios is the cohesive approach (Karlowicz 2000). A cohesive approach concurs with Knowles's view that evaluation should form a component of any self-directed learning activity. Similarly, a synthesis of learning within the portfolio is expected (Rassin *et al.* 2006). The portfolio should knit together so that both evidence and critical analysis weave together to form the overall account (Jasper 2006a). Within this section the relevant learning within the portfolio may be summarized and it may be ascertained whether or not personal learning goals are achieved. As Lyons (1998: 5) suggests, 'the real power of a portfolio process . . . may well be in the acts of . . . constructing, presenting and reflecting on the . . . evidence'. Proposals for the type of reflection that might be considered useful will now be discussed.

Selecting a model of reflection

Personalized self-reflection for personal self-development appears inadequate to fully interpret the meaning and extract relevant learning from practice that is required within your student portfolio. Without consideration of models of reflection that incorporate the wider social context, 'the portfolio, as a method of self-reflection, becomes a means to evaluate personal satisfaction and self-worth' (Wenzel *et al.* 1998: 210). This seems to be a common theme throughout student portfolio use. While there is certainly some merit in self-development, and clearly a portfolio sub-aim is personal development, its primary purpose is to display a cohesive account of work-based learning that contains relevant evidence from and critical reflection on practice. Klenowski (2002: 3) believes that a portfolio 'provides opportunities for students to self-evaluate their own growth' and similarly Mitchell (1994) equates self-reflection within the portfolio with increased student confidence and self-awareness. There are currently many who view this personalized approach to reflection as being of limited value, particularly in practice settings.

In order to address some of these concerns, it is important to select a model for use for reflection within the portfolio that is able to withstand challenges in relation to its validity. Two initial categories, used as criteria for assessing the potential rigour of models of reflection – explication of origins and comprehensiveness of content (Cormack and Reynolds 1992) – were discussed in Chapter 3 and will be alluded to briefly below. Logical congruence, generation of theory, and credibility of selected models will now be further discussed to support a more rigorous consideration of the selection of a framework for reflection.

In relation to comprehensiveness of content, critical theory is identified as having a useful contribution to make to the explication of the portfolio. However, while providing guiding principles for portfolio aims, it imparts little in terms of a comprehensive framework or actual tangible model that could be used to derive evidence for the portfolio. Habermas's (1971) work, for example, lacks specific (as opposed to philosophical) direction for enquiry (Swindall 1999). This means for you as a student it is difficult to pull out a tangible framework for use from this work. Other authors that use critical theory have developed models that would be overly complex for your use. For example, Kim (1999) used a three-phase critical theory approach (descriptive phase, reflective phase, critical/emancipatory phase) to analyse nurses' narratives on clinical experience. This is primarily a proposed research methodology (Kim 1999) and is too complex for use in practical settings (Rolfe *et al.* 2001). Others focus too much on the individualistic approach. Taylor (2000, 2006) uses Habermas's (1971) modes of enquiry, citing particular relevance for nursing practice. Thus she outlines a popular reflective framework that examines empirical (generated through the scientific method), interpretive (generated through understanding and lived experience) and critical (emancipatory, based in critical social theory) knowledge. While popular in nursing, this has primarily an individualistic approach (Rolfe *et al.* 2001), which limits its usefulness in practice. Furthermore, as it is intended for use in nursing practice situations, its approach is limited in terms of direction for comprehensive analysis, in the manner that might be required within your comprehensive portfolio. Taylor's (2000, 2006) framework for reflection is simplistic and consists primarily of a series of statements. The search for a comprehensive framework from within critical theory was thus limited. Barnett (1997) fared highly in Chapter 3 with regard to rigour both in relation to its origin and provision of the most comprehensive model of reflection, and you may find this model useful.

In terms of comprehensiveness, Barnett (1997) also offers a very thorough and far-reaching model that explores knowledge, self and the world. So rather than utilizing a model that focuses primarily on your descriptions and experience, Barnett moves the discussion outside of oneself to consider the wider world of practice. Boud and Walker (1990, 1993) also provide a very comprehensive and contemporary account of learning from experience and workplace learning, which has received a recent update (Boud *et al.* 2006). Framing your reflections as a student within the context of 'workplace learning' as suggested by Boud *et al.* (2006) is very useful and practical, as this is exactly what is taking place. Boud believes that valuable learning takes place in the practice domain, and reflection is a means to unlock this tacit learning.

Many models of reflection offer a checklist approach that is recognized by Boud and Walker (1993) to have limited value when an individual is engaged in learning from experience, as opposed to learning from one incident. A further limitation of many contemporary models is their 'verbalist' orientation

(Gitterman *et al.* 2004: 1186), implying a verbal or written exercise, rather than an action imperative. Boud and Walker (1993) are very critical of this evolution of reflective models posed as a series of questions and answers. This checklist format appears in many models of reflection (Borton 1970; Gibbs 1988; Johns 1999, 2004; Taylor 2000, 2006). Rolfe *et al.* (2001:35), for example, propose Borton's (1970) framework for reflection (What? So what? Now what?) and suggest that this and other frameworks provide mere 'cues' for reflection. This checklist approach in current use is possibly due to a primary focus on individual self-development within particular situations, rather than the broad focus of clinical experiences that your portfolio requires. In addition, when used for this specific purpose of personal development within practice, as most of these simplistic frameworks are, they act, as Rolfe *et al.* (2001) suggest, as cues for the practitioner rather than providing the comprehensive framework for critical reflection that may be required. From the review, Barnett (1997) puts forward the most comprehensive account of critical reflection whereas Boud and Walker (1990, 1993) provide a comprehensive and interesting account of learning from experience. A combination of approaches is proposed that would provide the most comprehensive model to satisfy many portfolio aims. Both Barnett (1997) and Boud and Walker (Boud and Walker 1990, 1993) are comprehensive models whose origins comply with the aims of a portfolio. In order to explore the rigour of these models further, to identify their suitability to the portfolio, their logical congruence will now be considered.

Logical congruence

Barnett's (1997) use of criticality within the domains of self, world and knowledge are useful as building blocks for reflection. Similarly, Boud and Walker's (1990, 1993) concept of learning from experience has particular resonance as students utilize the portfolio to draw out particular learning from a series of events during their programme. The aims of your portfolio require not just *self*-reflection, but rather a reflexive account of your contribution to knowledge and practice. While Boud and Walker's model offers the strongest position in terms of examining and learning from past experiences, a model encompassing greater reflexivity and critical reflection is required to investigate fully the context in which the learning takes place and actions arise.

Barnett (1997) proposes a framework of *criticality* with broader application to practice beyond self-development. The only direct application of Barnett's *et al.*'s work within health care was located in Brechin *et al.*'s book on critical practice (Brechin 2000). However, his numerous writings on the subject of knowledge within higher education are widely cited. Barnett (1997) describes reflection as a component of a broader concept of critical thought. Barnett provides the important components of critical theory that are essential to portfolio use: reflexive knowledge, the search for meaning and understanding as a legitimate form of enquiry and the importance of context. Barnett (1997) concurs with Habermas's (1971) view that knowledge is socially constructed. Rather than focusing on individual learning, Barnett emphasizes the importance, within disciplines, of broadening out the narrow lens of critical thinking or reflection, to a more inclusive, collaborative model of critical thought. Ultimately, Barnett suggests that disciplines require not only critical self-reflection but also critical analysis and action. He describes three classifications of 'criticality' which together outline the '*scope* of critical being' (Barnett 1997: 69) (emphasis author's own). These are critical reason, critical self-reflection and critical action. These operate within what Barnett describes as the domains of criticality – knowledge, self and the world (Table 6.1). Barnett (1997) suggests that criticality within the three domains of knowledge, self and the world together overlap to produce the critical person or being (Figure 6.1). Through the use of criticality within the three domains the person deploys *criticality frameworks in action* and professional knowledge becomes 'critique in action' (Barnett 1997: 139). The person therefore becomes a *critical being* concerned with critical self-reflection, critical action and critical reason (Barnett 1997).

Critical reason

Within the domain of knowledge, Barnett (1997) describes the application of forms of criticality as critical *reason* (Table 6.1). This suggests critical thought with regard to 'propositions, ideas and theories, especially as they are proffered in the world of systematic knowledge' (Barnett 1997: 65). It involves the questioning of established doctrine, policies, procedures and knowledge using critical thinking skills. Within the knowledge domain, overarching skills of self-reflection are utilized across the levels of criticality. Thus self-reflection is not confined to the domain of self, but essential self-reflective skills are required across all domains. Critical reason encompasses self-reflection of a disciplinary and educational nature and begins with critical thinking skills within the discipline. It then moves on to reflexivity, which incorporates reflection and challenging of one's own understanding. After this begins the refashioning of understandings by critical thought regarding assumptions of the discipline and finally transformation occurs in this area through formal critique of knowledge. *Critical reason* occurs exclusively within the domain of *knowledge*.

Table 6.1 The three domains of the critical being and their associated forms of criticality

Domains	Forms of criticality
1 Knowledge	Critical reason
2 Self	Critical self-reflection
3 World	Critical action

Source: Barnett (1997).

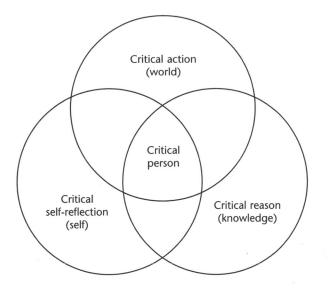

Figure 6.1 The critical being as an integration of the three forms of criticality

Source: Adapted from Barnett (1997).

Critical self-reflection

Critical self-reflection encompasses reflection that is critically reflective and ultimately involves self-realization. This commences with the use of critical thinking skills within the discipline in the form of self-monitoring according to required standards and norms. It then progresses to reflexivity incorporating reflection on one's own work. Subsequently, the refashioning of understandings through the development of self within traditions and finally transformation occurs through reconstruction of self. *Critical* self-reflection occurs wholly in the domain of self. What is interesting about this conceptualization is that it moves beyond the standard 'how do I feel' about situations, towards an examination of your knowledge on a topic in relation to the knowledge of the discipline, and a comparison of your behaviour in relation to standards in the practice discipline. If, from the earlier example, you were to reflect upon your actions in relation to communicating with a patient, in the domain of self, you would begin to consider more than just how you thought and felt about a situation, and what you may do differently (which is ultimately self-limiting) towards consideration of the knowledge base that informed your practice and how your skills and behaviours compared with an expert nurse.

Critical action

Critical action occurs in the world, that is, in the practice environment. Barnett (1997) emphasizes the 'world' as the most crucial and neglected area of reflection. He believes criticality needs to be emphasized here in relation to the practice environment. He describes the domain of the world as the 'dominant mode(s) of reflection'. Barnett (1997: 99) believes strongly that the self-reflection of metacompetence (reflection on competence and skills within the discipline), reflective practice and active problem solving used within this domain could act as a 'self-monitoring of one's performance in the real world' and ultimately improve the practice of the discipline.

Barnett (1997) asserts that up until now, criticality has been marginally interpreted, relying only upon reflection in the formal knowledge domain: 'critical being in the other two domains of self and of the world, has, until recently, been neglected; in so far as they have been given any attention, critical self-reflection and critical action have been accorded a marginal place' (Barnett 1997: 77). He suggests that criticality should include a framework for critical action thereby facilitating decision-making and action in the real world of practice. Interestingly, students view action, in the form of personal behaviour change, as an essential outcome of reflection (Shields 1995). Critical action, Barnett suggests, involves four feats: critical skills, reflexivity, refashioning of traditions and transformatory critique.

Rather than merely reflecting internally on events (at a personal level), these classifications of criticality allow individuals to act as critical beings. Thus, not only reflecting and thinking critically within oneself, this self-reflection is extended to critical analysis of knowledge that informs practice and also extends to critical action within the world. So Barnett's (1997: 70) classification of criticality extends beyond reflection and allows the individual to 'act critically in the wider world, or to evaluate critically theories produced within bodies of thought or, indeed, to understand (oneself) critically'. From your perspective as a student, this may involve you sharing your views with regard to potential actions with your facilitator, or perhaps performing future literature reviewing or research on a topic, for example nurse–patient communication, that you may then be able to feed back to the practice environment.

Rather than a self-limiting personalized descriptive narrative, an explicit framework such as Barnett's (1997) provides a rigorous framework that provides more specific and detailed responses to your own personal interrogation. Rather than simply to introspect, or reflect on your past actions, this framework provides for reflexivity. Reflexivity provides for a deeper analysis that goes 'beyond the usual introspective focus of reflection to consider the wider social and political context' (Freshwater and Rolfe 2001: 530). It allows students to analyse previously held beliefs, question the impetus for actions and consider the outcomes. This provides new meanings and understandings, which is the very essence of the portfolio, thus providing an 'understanding of self in context' (Freshwater and Rolfe 2001: 531). From your reflections on your communication skills, for example, you may have noticed that you raised your voice when speaking with an elderly client, without considering other non-verbal approaches that could have been used. From a social perspective, your reading within the discipline may indicate to you that the elderly are often a marginalized group, which in a sense your behaviours compounded. This new and additional information can improve and alter your future practice and perhaps that of the health care environment, if you are encouraged to share your reflections.

Although opposed to formulaic approaches, Freshwater and Avis (2004) suggest that critical reflection, as a method, should use structured processes. Therefore the development of a specific framework for critical reflection, using Barnett's (1997) work, allows for interpretation on your practice as a student that 'sheds new light on the meaning' (Freshwater and Avis 2004:9). A preliminary framework is presented in Table 6.2. Table 6.2 outlines the emerging framework for critical reflection based on application and interpretation of Barnett's (1997) work.

The consideration of reflection within the three domains: knowledge, self, and world, together with the reflexive approach and overt consideration of context indicate logical congruence with the aim of the portfolio. The framework also provides guidance to individuals with regard to its use and indicates the desired outcome (Cormack and Reynolds 1992). Within the domains of self, world and knowledge, specific guidance is provided about the nature of reflection within each. Different levels of criticality that can occur in each domain are outlined.

The emerging framework is descriptive and explanatory rather than providing a mechanism for operation. To this end, direction is required with regard to the reflection required. Boud and Walker's (1990, 1993) model provides the required synergism. Barnett (1997) provides the consideration of context and environment lacking in Boud and Walker (but recognized by them as

Table 6.2 An emerging framework for reflection 1

Critical reason	Discipline-specific critical thinking skills
	Critical thinking (reflecting on ones own understanding)
	Critical thought (regarding traditions of thought)
	Knowledge critique
Critical self-reflection	Self-monitoring to given standards and norms
	Self-reflection (reflection on ones own projects)
	Development of self within traditions
	Reconstruction of self
Critical action	Problem-solving
	Reflective practice (adaptability; flexibility)
	Mutual understanding and development of traditions
	Critique-in-action (collective reconstruction of world)

Source: Barnett (1997).

important) Walker, whereas Boud and Walker provide a detailed model for looking back, interpreting experiences and learning from these. By super-imposing Boud and Walker's model onto Barnett's framework, a useable framework emerges (Table 6.3).

Further consistencies with the use of Boud and Walker (1990, 1993) include a focus on overall learning from experience being thereby compatible with the aim of your portfolio. This model provides for you to learn more from *experience* than from reflection in order to develop a new understanding and appreciation. The first phase is *returning* to the experience. Boud and Walker's model also attempts to deal with feelings *associated* with the event. Rather than actually drawing too much inference from what these feelings mean, it suggests that you pay attention to how you were feeling at the time, or how you feel thinking back on it. It is rather paying attention to the feelings described as *attending to the feeling*. Boud and Walker are cognizant that feelings emerge from a personal perspective, and don't necessarily reflect or interpret the reality of the event. The following stages of the model serve to evaluate these feelings and put them into perspective.

The next phase, *re-evaluating the experience*, is further broken down into three stages:

1 Association, whereby new information from the reflection is associated with existing knowledge and attitudes and the relationships are observed.

TABLE 6.3 An emerging framework for reflection 2

Critical reason	Discipline-specific Critical thinking skills Critical thinking (reflecting on ones own understanding) Critical thought (regarding traditions of thought) Knowledge critique	
Critical self-reflection	Self-monitoring to given standards and norms Self-reflection (reflection on ones won projects) Development of self within traditions Reconstruction of self	• Returning to the experience • Attending to the feeling • Association • Integration • Validation and appropriation
Critical action	Reflective practice (adaptability; flexibility) Mutual understanding and development of traditions Critique-in-action (collective reconstruction of world)	

Source: Boud and Walker (1990, 1993) Barnett (1997).

2 Integration: identifying the nature of the relationships that have been observed in the association phase and drawing new conclusions and insights from the data towards the piecing together of new attitudes.
3 These are then tested by validation to ascertain whether there are contradictions or inconsistencies between the new understandings and existing knowledge and beliefs.

Boud and Walker (1990: 61)

Again the terminology here is very fitting. The aim of a portfolio is to develop knowledge in a work-based setting: in the particular social and personal context in which it occurred. Outcomes expressed by other models are restrictive, relying on questions such as 'what would you do if it happened again?' (Gibbs 1988) and 'How do I now feel about this experience?' (Johns 1999, 2004). Boud and Walker allow students to make sense of this reflection by seeing where it fits with new knowledge that may have developed and is ultimately focused on learning from experience that is simply personal and introspective. Boud and Walker (1998) pay particular attention to the social construction of knowledge and the limits of personal approaches to reflection. A facilitator is suggested to support your reflection and assist with the phases of association and evaluation.

Moreover, the authors have recently moved away from the use of specific frameworks of reflection (Boud and Walker 1998) to a broader concept of experience-based learning (EBL) (Andresen *et al.* 2000; Boud *et al.* 2006). Within this concept, the authors encourage learning from experience based on the guiding principles that learning is socially and culturally constructed and influenced by the socio-economic context in which it occurs (Boud and Walker 1993). For these authors, reflection still holds a central place within EBL, but this is only one component of a broader concept of learning from experience (Andresen *et al.* 2000). These authors still value their model of enquiry (Boud *et al.* 1985; Boud and Walker 1990, 1993) as facilitative while learning from experience but accept that this requires additional consideration of context and culture. However, they do not provide specific direction with regard to this and admit that 'there is no adequate framework to assist learners to promote learning in the midst of experience' (Boud and Walker 1990: 61). So ultimately there remains a great deal of flexibility with regard to the model of choice. It is the end goal of knowledge development and learning from experience that is important.

Credibility

Fawcett (1995) suggests that credibility of conceptual models requires consideration. In terms of specific questions to direct this particular enquiry, Cormack and Reynolds (1992) suggest questioning whether the model is based on tested and accepted theory and whether it is valid and reliable? It is useful to consider current criticisms of reflection. A critique of reflective practice

(Carroll *et al.* 2002) suggests that further empirical work is required to identify the ultimate benefits of reflection and reflective practice to practice and patient care. Carroll *et al.* (2002) suggest that while reflection is a useful tool for learning, they are sceptical about its evidence base. These views are supported by Newell (2002), who previously voiced scepticism with regard to the proposed benefits of reflection for these reasons (Newell 1994). However, Rolfe (2005) contests these arguments, suggesting that the reflection itself provides the empirical evidence.

The two models of reflection that emerge strongly from an analysis of origins, comprehensiveness and logical congruence, Boud and Walker (1990, 1993) and Barnett (1997), certainly have sufficient theoretical detail to provide for rigorous examination. Barnett drew extensively on the work of Habermas (1971), Foucault (1974, 1980) and Popper (1972). However, whereas Habermas's (1971) work lacks specific direction for reflection on action (Swindall 1999), Barnett's (1997) work provides a practical application of critical social theory, suitable for use within disciplines (Brechin 2000), thus providing a claim to credibility. Boud *et al.*'s (1985) model underwent significant development over a twenty-year period (Boud and Walker 1990, 1993, 1998; Andresen *et al.* 2000). Their work has developed from their teaching and workshops in Sydney, Australia, and from their international writings and presentation. Their recent book demonstrates significant theoretical development as their work formed the basis of a large longitudinal international research project entitled *Productive Reflection at Work* (Boud *et al.* 2006).

In terms of credibility, two prominent academics, McKenna (1999) and Yoong (1999) recommend Boud *et al.*'s (1985) model for use in development of practice theory. This support for its use, together with the level of conceptual development, lends credibility and validity to this model, thus rendering it suitable for inclusion. Similarly, Barnett (1997) has also been understood and simply applied to health and social care practice by Brechin (2000). Although no specific testing of the latter framework has been identified, its subsequent adaptation by Brechin (2000) provides quite detailed application within health and social care. Furthermore, this publication of Barnett's (1997) work as a contemporary model of reflection for practitioners in health and social care is a testament to its reliability and validity. This level of testing may suffice, and is certainly comparable to a limited level of testing of other models of reflection (Carroll *et al.* 2002). It also complies with Rolfe's (2005) notion that the interpretive application suffices for reflection; rigorous testing, he suggested, is not required. In addition to credibility, theory generation is also a consideration when selecting appropriate models (Fawcett 1995).

Generation of theory

Barnett's (1997) work is certainly comprehensive, logical, congruent and credible (Brechin 2000). Theory generation potential is also present. It was directed at professionals working in disciplines and from this perspective is ultimately congruent with the portfolio aims. Similarly, Boud and Walker (1990, 1993), through their recent international research initiatives (Boud *et al.* 2006), continue to generate theory. There is also potential for theory generation demonstrated through the application of these frameworks to a student portfolio. As previously described, the individualistic, simplistic and situation-focused nature of most models of reflection renders it difficult to generate theory that can be applied outside the individual (Boud and Walker 1990, 1993).

Given the consistency of Barnett's (1997) and Boud and Walker's (1990, 1993) frameworks with the overall portfolio aims, and their comprehensiveness, credibility and potential for theory generation, this combined approach offers a novel and applicable approach to reflection that has logical congruence with a portfolio. In practical application of Barnett's proposed framework it is useful to consider Brechin's (2000) synthesis of this model. Brechin further develops Barnett's (1997) seminal ideas for use in the health care context. Brechin expands and builds upon Barnett's framework of criticality and suggests that criticality (termed critical practice by Brechin) is an essential component of contemporary health care. Brechin (2000) recognizes the value of criticality for contemporary health and social care. She recommends that health care workers operate within the criticality framework and termed this *critical practice*. Through adaptation of Barnett's original work (1997) the three classifications of critical practice (critical reason, critical self-reflection and critical action) were further described as 'domains' of critical analysis, critical reflexivity and critical action (Figure 6.2).

Brechin's (2000) interpretation of Barnett's (1997) framework is both innovative and original. The language and simplicity that Brechin applied was useful and practical in a professional sense. Her use of the term critical analysis (rather than critical reason) and critical reflexivity (rather than critical reflection) may have more practical application and resonance with nursing students than the original interpretation. Furthermore, her extrapolation of the essence of critical practice, as the overlap of this model, is very user-friendly, rather than the term critical being as applied by Barnett. Using Barnett's original work, adapted by Brechin (2000), a final framework emerges that may be used to support entries within the portfolio in a more cohesive way than some contemporary models (Table 6.4). In the first phase, critical analysis, both technical and empirical knowledge related to the performance indicator may be outlined, perhaps by including and evaluating (through discussion) research articles, policies or guidelines. Critical reflexivity involves engaging oneself in critical reflection, keeping the context of the wider practice environment in mind. Boud and Walker's (1990, 1993) model may be further used here to support personal reflection. In the final phase, critical action, future or present actions based on learning from practice may be outlined.

A comprehensive approach to reflection, such as is suggested, within the portfolio is useful to move reflection from personal introspection to more meaningful learning that contributes ultimately to practice: 'The portfolio

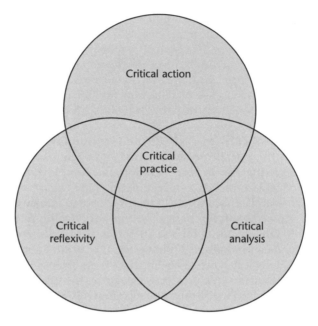

Figure 6.2 Three overlapping domains of critical analysis, critical reflexivity and critical action

Source: Brechin (2000).

needs to demonstrate a critical attitude towards the student's own practice . . . The portfolio also needs to capture the student's ability to identify alternative ways of practice and envisage strategies for change' (Joyce 2005: 460), suggesting perhaps a more critical approach. Ultimately there are a range of models available for use in reflection that are well described in books on the topic and in books that address reflection in relation to portfolio use (Pearce 2003). The selection and the manner of selection proposed in this chapter is a guide only, and Jasper (2006b) further suggests a framework for selection (Box 6.9). This selection process permits you to select a framework or model of reflection (if there is choice available) according to your needs.

Evaluation

Regardless of the model of reflection either personally chosen or recommended by your Nursing School, according to our guiding principles for self-directed learning and attending to learning needs (Table 1.2), evaluation of learning within the portfolio process model is a key feature in developing the cohesive portfolio. Ask yourself what you have achieved through developing the portfolio? Look back and examine whether you achieved the set learning objectives? And if not, why not?

Table 6.4 A final framework for critical reflection within the portfolio

Critical analysis	Evaluation of knowledge, theories, policy, and practice Recognition of multiple perspectives Different levels of analysis Ongoing enquiry	
Critical reflexivity	Engaged self Self-monitoring to given standards and norms Negotiated understanding Questioning personal values and assumptions	• Returning to the experience • Attending to the feeling • Association • Integration • Validation and appropriation
Critical action	Sound skill base used with awareness of context Mutual understanding Problem-solving	

Source: Boud and Walker (1990, 1993) Barnett (1997) Brechin (2000).

Box 6.9 Criteria for selecting a framework for reflection within the portfolio

- What am I trying to achieve?
- How do I want to reflect?
- Who do I want to reflect with?
- What sort of structure do I want to sue?
- When do I want to reflect?
- What are the values underpinning and inherent to the model?
- How do these fit with my own values as a practitioner?

Source: Jasper (2006b).

Conclusion

One challenge of portfolio completion is its time-consuming nature (Murray 1994). It can also be difficult to put a word limit on a portfolio that is being submitted for assessment purposes due to the uniqueness of each one (Pearce 2003).

It is useful to break the portfolio down into component parts such as 'entries' – individual discussions on areas of practice related to competencies or learning outcomes. Care needs to be taken, however, when the portfolio is broken down by subsections in this way, that a dialogue is maintained throughout sections (Pearce 2003; Endacott *et al.* 2004). Through use of relevant subheadings and a comprehensive model of reflection it is possible to prepare a cohesive and meaningful portfolio that will enhance your practice experience and enable you to gain valuable learning from your practice experiences.

Summary of key points

- Evidence in the portfolio is crucial and helps to support claims that you are making.
- The portfolio may take one of two common forms: either a competency-based portfolio, used in conjunction with the curriculum to provide for appropriate assessment of clinical performance, or a negotiated learning portfolio, which involves negotiating specific learning outcomes.
- Following clear guidelines with regard to the portfolio development is useful.
- Unless otherwise stated, a framework for reflection may be selected based upon specific purpose.

References

An Bord Altranais (2004) *Requirements and Standards for Nurse Registration Education Programmes*. Dublin: An Bord Altranais.

Andresen, L., Boud, D. *et al.* (2000) Experience-based learning, in G. Foley (ed.) *Understanding Adult Education and Training*. Sydney: Allen & Unwin.

Barnett, R. (1997) *Higher Education: A Critical Business*. Bristol: Society for Research into Higher Education.

Baumard, P. (1999) *Tacit Knowledge in Organizations*. London: Sage Publications.

Borton, T. (1970) *Reach, Touch and Teach*. London: McGraw-Hill.

Boud, D., Cressey, P. *et al.* (2006) Setting the scene for productive reflection at work, in D. Boud, P. Cressey and P. Doherty (eds) *Productive Reflection at Work*. Oxford: Routledge.

Boud, D., Keogh, R. *et al.* (1985) Promoting reflection in learning: a model, in D. Boud, D. Walker and R. Keogh (eds) *Reflection: Turning Experience into Learning*. London: Kogan Page.

Boud, D. and Walker, D. (1990) Making the most of experience, *Studies in Continuing Education*, 12(2): 61–80.

Boud, D. and Walker, D. (1993) Barriers to reflection on experience, in D. Boud, R. Cohen and D. Walker (eds) *Using Experience For Learning*. Buckingham: Society for Research into Higher Education and Open University Press.

Boud, D. and Walker, D. (1998) Promoting reflection in professional courses: the challenge of context, *Studies in Higher Education*, 23(2): 191–207.

Brechin, A. (2000) Introducing critical practice, in A. Brechin, H. Brown and E. M. London (eds) *Critical Practice in Health and Social Care*. London: Sage Publications.

Calman, L., Watson, R. *et al.* (2002) Assessing practice of student nurses: methods, preparation of assessors and student views, *Journal of Advanced Nursing*, 38(5): 516–23.

Carroll, M., Curtis, L. *et al.* (2002) Is there a place for reflective practice in the nursing curriculum?, *Nurse Education in Practice*, 2(1): 13–20.

Coffey, A. (2005) The clinical learning portfolio: a practice development experience in gerontological nursing, *Journal of Clinical Nursing*, 14(2): 75–83.

Cooper, T. (1999) *Portfolio Assessment: A Guide for Lecturers, Teachers and Course Designers*. Perth: Praxis Education.

Corcoran, J. and Nicholson, C. (2004) Learning portfolios – evidence of learning: an examination of students' perspectives, *Nursing in Critical Care*, 9(5): 230–7.

Cormack, D. F. S. and Reynolds, W. (1992) Criteria for evaluating the clinical and practical utility of models used by nurses, *Journal of Advanced Nursing*, 17(12): 1472–8.

Dolan, G. (2003) Assessing student nurse clinical competency: will we ever get it right?, *Journal of Clinical Nursing*, 12(1): 132–41.

Dolan, G., Fairbairn, G. *et al.* (2004) Is our student portfolio valued?, *Nurse Education Today*, 24(1): 4–13.

Emden, C., Hutt, D. *et al.* (2003) Exemplar: Portfolio learning/assessment in nursing and midwifery: an innovation in progress, *Contemporary Nurse*, 16(1–2): 124–32.

Endacott, R., Gray, M. A. *et al.* (2004) Using portfolios in the assessment of learning and competence: the impact of four models, *Nurse Education in Practice*, 4(4): 250–7.

Fawcett, J. (1995) *Analysis and Evaluation of Conceptual Models of Nursing*. Philadelphia, PA: FA Davis.

Foucault, M. (1974) *The Archaelogy of Knowledge*. London: Tavistock.

Foucault, M. (1980) *Power/Knowledge*. Hemel Hemstead: Harvester Wheatsheaf.

Freshwater, D. and Avis, M. (2004) Analysing interpretation and reinterpreting analysis: exploring the logic of critical reflection, *Nursing Philosophy*, 5: 4–11.

Freshwater, D. and Rolfe, G. (2001) Critical reflexivity: a politically and ethically engaged research method for nursing, *NTResearch*, 6(1): 526–38.

Gallagher, P. (2001) An evaluation of a standards based portfolio [corrected and republished article originally printed in *Nurse Education Today*, 21(3), April 2001: 197–200].

Gibbs, G. (1988) *Learning by Doing: A Guide to Teaching Learning Methods*. Oxford: Oxford Brookes University.

Gitterman, D. P., Greenwood, R. S. *et al.* (2004) Did a rising tide lift all boats? The NIH budget and pediatric research portfolio, *Health Affairs*, 23(5): 113–24.

Griffin, C. (2001) *The Development of Competencies for Registration*. Assessment of Competence Conference. Dublin: An Bord Altranais.

Habermas, J. (1971) Knowledge and human interests, translated by J. J. Shapiro. Boston: Beacon.

Harris, S., Dolan, G. *et al.* (2001) Reflecting on the use of student portfolios, *Nurse Education Today*, 21(4): 278–86.

Jasper, M. (2006a) Portfolios and the use of evidence, in M. Jasper (ed.) *Professional Development, Reflection and Decision Making*. Oxford: Blackwell Publishing 154–183.

Jasper, M. (2006b) Reflection and reflective practice, in M. Jasper (ed.) *Professional Development, Reflection and Decision Making*. Oxford: Blackwell Publishing 39–80.

Johns, C. (1999) *Becoming a Reflective Practitioner*. Oxford: Blackwell.

Johns, C. (2004) *Becoming a Reflective Practitioner*, 2nd edn. Oxford: Blackwell.

Joyce, P. (2005) A framework for portfolio development in postgraduate nursing practice, *Journal of Clinical Nursing*, 14(4): 456–63.

Karlowicz, K. A. (2000) The value of student portfolios to evaluate undergraduate nursing programs, *Nurse Educator*, 25(2): 82–7.

Kim, H. S. (1999) Critical reflective inquiry for knowledge development in nursing practice, *Journal of Advanced Nursing*, 29(5): 1205–12.

Klenowski, V. (2002) *Developing Portfolios for Learning and Assessment: Processes and Principles*. Oxford: Routledge.

Knowles, M., Holton, E. *et al.* (1998) *The Adult Learner: The Definitive Classic in Adult Education and Human Resource Development*, 5th edn. Houston, TX: Gulf Publishing.

Knowles, M. S. (1989) *The Adult Learner: A Neglected Species*. Houston, TX: Gulf Publishing.

Lyons, N. (1998) *With Portfolio in Hand. Validating the New Teacher Professionalism*. New York: Teachers College Press.

McKenna, H. (1999) The role of reflection in the development of practice theory: a case study, *Journal of Psychiatric and Mental Health Nursing*, 6: 147–51.

McMullan, M., Endacott, R. *et al.* (2003) Portfolios and assessment of competence: a review of the literature, *Journal of Advanced Nursing*, 41(3): 283–94.

Mitchell, M. (1994) The views of students and teachers on the use of portfolios as a learning and assessment tool in midwifery education, *Nurse Education Today*, 14(1): 38–43.

Murray, P. J. (1994) Portfolios and accreditation of prior experiential learning (APEL) make credits . . . or problems? *Nurse Education Today*, 14(3): 232–7.

Murrell, K., Harris, L. *et al.* (1998) Using a portfolio to assess clinical practice, *Professional Nurse*, 13(4): 220–3.

Newell, R. (1994) Reflection: art, science or pseudo-science, *Nurse Education Today*, 14: 79–81.

Newell, R. (2002) Commentary on Carroll, M., Curtis, L., Higgins, A., Nicholl, H., Redmond, R., Timmins, F. 'Is there a place for reflection in the nursing curriculum?', *Clinical Effectiveness in Nursing*, 6(1): 42–3.

NMC (2004) Standards of Proficiency for Pre-registration Nursing Education. London: Nursing and Midwifery Council.

Pearce, R. (2003) *Profiles and Portfolios of Evidence*. Cheltenham: Nelson Thornes.

Popper, K. (1972) *Objective Knowledge*. Oxford: Oxford University Press.

Price, B. (2003) Building a portfolio: professional gains, *Nursing Standard*, 17(48): 32–33.

Rassin, M., Silner, D. *et al.* (2006) Departmental portfolio in nursing – an advanced instrument, *Nurse Education in Practice*, 6(1): 55–60.

Rolfe, G. (2005) The deconstructing angel: nursing, reflection and evidence-based practice, *Nursing Inquiry*, 12(2): 78–86.

Rolfe, G., Freshwater, D. *et al.* (2001) *Critical Reflection for Nursing and the Helping Professions: A User's Guide*. Basingstoke: Palgrave.

Serembus, J. F. (2000) Teaching the process of developing a professional portfolio, *Nurse Educator*, 25(6): 282–7.

Sherrod, D. (2005) Career scope: south Atlantic. The professional portfolio: a snapshot of your career, *Nursing Management*, 36(9): 74–5.

Shields, E. (1995) Reflection and learning in student nurses, *Nurse Education Today*, 15(452): 8.

Storey, L. and Haigh C. (2002) Portfolios in professional practice, *Nurse Education in Practice*, 2(1): 44–8.

Swindall, J. (1999) *Reflection Revisited: Jürgen Habermas's Discursive Theory of Truth.* New York: Fordham University Press.

Taylor, B. (2000) *Reflective Practice: A Guide for Nurses and Midwives.* Buckingham: Open University Press.

Taylor, B. (2006) *Reflective Practice: A Guide for Nurses and Midwives*, 2nd edn. Buckingham: Open University Press.

Turner, D. S. and Beddoes, L. (2007) Using reflective models to enhance learning: experiences of staff and students, *Nurse Education in Practice*, 7(3): 135–40.

Wenzel, L. S., Briggs, K. L. *et al.* (1998) Portfolio: authentic assessment in the age of the curriculum revolution, *Journal of Nursing Education*, 37(5): 209–12.

Williams, M. (2003) Developing portfolios for peri-operative nurses, *Nursing Standard*, 18(1): 46–54.

Yoong, P. (1999) Making sense of group support systems facilitation: a reflective practice perspective, *Information Technology & People*, 12(1): 86–112.

7

The Portfolio in Operation

Fiona Timmins

Introduction • Working with a mentor • Working with your mentor to put the portfolio together • Gathering the evidence • Conclusion • Summary of key points • References

Introduction

The nursing student portfolio that you are most likely to complete requires you to fill a receptacle, such as a handheld ring binder, with appropriate evidence from practice. It can also take the form of a handheld electronic device. Very often, you, as a student, carry this portfolio and you prepare and complete it while you are actually gaining your practical experience within the clinical practice environment. As discussed in previous chapters, this portfolio may be used in part, or indeed in full, to support the assessment of your clinical competence by a registered nurse or it may be used in a more specific way that is designed to achieve particular learning outcomes. The approach to its use varies considerably between Nursing Schools. Using a receptacle (such as a ring binder/electronic device) is the easy part; knowing exactly what to put in the portfolio and how to operate a portfolio is another matter entirely! Absence of, or lack of clarity regarding guidelines, overt freedom and choice with regard to structure, lack of formal assessment or grade, lack of substantial student preparation and failure of students to attach significance to the portfolio are but some of the reasons why you may find putting the portfolio together a daunting task. Building on the information from contemporary literature that has been unpacked in previous chapters, this chapter aims to provide some information and advice about putting the portfolio into practice. The registered nurse who is your mentor or facilitator in the clinical area has a vital role to play in this operation and this will be further explored (Farrell 2004; Hull *et al.* 2005). Recent attempts to conceptualize understandings of supervision processes for nursing students from an international perspective refer solely to the term mentor, despite an apparent multiplicity of terms (Fulton *et al.* 2007) For the purposes of this discussion, the supportive facilitator of the portfolio will be referred to as a mentor.

Working with a mentor

Portfolio use is firmly rooted in the context of adult and student-centred learning (Chapter 1). In keeping with this philosophical stance, nursing students preparing a portfolio ought to demonstrate independence but also ideally require a facilitator who will support them to develop ways of independent learning. As we discovered in Chapter 1, facilitation is a key concept in adult learning and, through the use of certain behaviours and creation of an appropriate environment, you as a student are encouraged by the mentor to become more active in your own learning. This applies to your learning across the clinical environment but, in this particular context, to the portfolio. Facilitation could be considered the second half of the self-directed learning equation. You have at least some ability to learn independently, and the mentor, by creating an appropriate environment, fosters this independent learning. It is important to remember this term *facilitation* as we proceed through the chapter. You may be familiar with this term in relation to your mentor in the clinical area.

> **Remember!**
> The self-directed learning equation: student effort + facilitation = independent learning.

Many students today are familiar with working with a mentor; this function denotes a 'formal supervisory role and is used to describe the role of a qualified nurse who facilitates learning and supervises students in the practice setting' (Saarikoski *et al.* 2007). In many situations, this mentor position is formalized and understood throughout the health care system, and this is more advantageous to you as a student as, first, there is an onus on this registered nurse to support you in your learning and second, this nurse will have been prepared to take on the tasks that the role requires (Hull *et al.* 2005). Supervision of your clinical practice and facilitation of your learning are identified as core components of this mentor role.

Activity 1

Think about one of your learning experiences in the clinical area.

In what way was this learning facilitated by a registered nurse?

Can you identify behaviours of this mentor that positively contributed to your learning?

Write down your responses before proceeding with the chapter.

When you first present your portfolio to your mentor for advice, you could be met with an uncertainty on the part of the registered nurse that you may not have hitherto expected. As previously mentioned, ideally mentors are well prepared for their supportive and supervisory role in student learning, so therefore it may come as a surprise that they don't have all the answers. However, registered nurses' sometimes reticent approach can stem from the varied and individualized approach that each student portfolio can take, and the resultant absence of a clearly defined template that such a varied and individualistic task heralds. In a sense, to expect the mentor to 'tell you how' is a high expectation in this context. Furthermore, mentors are likely to face the same lack of clarity as you. If guidelines are broad and open to interpretation, the mentor is as much at a loss as you are. Mentors who have prepared their own portfolios in the recent past, as students, may be at some advantage, but with the nursing student portfolio currently standing as a somewhat nebulous concept, providing specific direction may prove difficult. However, it may be important to rethink your understanding of the role of a mentor. The notion of *teaching* is notably absent from the above definition. They are required to *supervise* you as you attend to or take part in patient care, and to facilitate your learning. Facilitation as we understand from Chapter 1 is about the mentor giving of themselves personally to you. This involves them being genuine, respectful, understanding and journeying with the student to reach required goals. This definition does not provide for telling you what to do with your portfolio, but rather it opens the door for a dialogue and discovery between you and your mentor. Farrell's (2004) study very clearly outlined this cooperative journey in which mentors were in the habit of 'going though' the nursing students' portfolios with them on a regular basis. They found this a very useful process and through this they came to understand where the students were in relation to their learning. One mentor said: 'You need to go through it [the portfolio] [then] there's more discussion' (Farrell 2004). They also highlighted that students develop primarily through their own effort.

It was also very clear from Farrell (2004) that the mentors held the nursing students in high esteem, and they respected their efforts and achievements in relation to their portfolios. These observations epitomize the facilitation relationship. The relationship is also about mutual respect (Andrews and Wallis 1999); this means, rather than disparaging a mentor who doesn't appear at first to understand what is required of you in the portfolio, you respect this individual's competence and expertise in his or her profession and accept his or her position. Mentors are a tremendous resource that can help you to link theory to practice, a fundamental principle in relation to operating the portfolio (Lambert and Glacken 2004). Mentors enjoy supporting students with their portfolios and find it a learning experience.

Remember!

Facilitation involves the mentor being genuine, respectful, understanding and journeying with you as a student to reach required goals. It also means mutuality with regard to these attributes.

Mentor support is viewed as crucial to students developing portfolios and, in the absence of such a facilitator, students can struggle with portfolio completion (O'Donovan 2006). Students also reveal that having a mentor gives them confidence.

Even though in some cases you as a student are really keen to receive direction about your portfolio from the mentor, it is essential that the mentor creates an environment that encourages your freedom and individuality (Rogers 1969, 1983). This environment occurs mostly within the relationship that develops, and this partnership can be crucial to success. Interestingly, students find that they like to be allowed to take this responsibility, although it is initially daunting as they begin to use their own initiative and work independently (Hamill 1995). This gives you the feeling of control over your learning. However, it is noted that students don't like excessive 'do it yourself' approaches (Hamill 1995), but rather require the supportive facilitation of a mentorship relationship.

Activity 2

Think about the way in which you like to learn. Do you agree with the students in Hamill's (1995) study with regard to 'do it yourself' approaches?

What aspects of this approach, if any, would you dislike?

Write down your views.

Familiarity rather than expertise with the portfolio is a requirement of your mentor. It is rather mentor *characteristics* as opposed to a specialized knowledge base in relation to particular teaching methods that contributes to your overall learning from this process (Andrews and Wallis 1999). Students respect mentors who appear to have good clinical nursing knowledge and skills, who are friendly and approachable and who have a good sense of humour. Characteristics of a 'good' mentor also include effective communication skills, a positive teaching style, paying attention to the need for a student to learn and providing supervisory support (Andrews and Wallis 1999).

These characteristics in mentors also serve to support you as a student when you feel that the portfolio as an assessment is a stressor. Mentors need to be mindful of assessments as potentially huge student stressors (Thyer and Bazeley 1993; Hamill 1995; Rhead 1995; Mahat 1996; Lindop 1999; Jones and Johnston 2000) and, moreover, continue the relationship in a facilitative style that supports students rather than burdens them, as this facilitation relationship can itself become a source of stress (Mahat 1996). Clearly negative behaviours such as overt criticism of students (Cavanagh and Snape 1997) may lead to students feeling negative and should be avoided.

The mentor/student relationship may proceed through a series of stages. Although the term relationship is used, and some suggest that this could be quite personal and emotional (May *et al.* 1982), it is essentially a professional relationship that occurs in the context of the working environment. Indeed, students describe this relationship as both 'supportive and professional' (Higgins and McCarthy 2005). Particular phases of the relationship are outlined as, first, an initial getting to know each other phase, as both parties begin to settle into the relationship (Andrews and Wallis 1999). So don't be at all surprised if you are a little nervous or unsettled around this new venture initially. This settles down as the relationship becomes more relaxed and open. A 'protégé' stage may develop, described as the peak time within the relationship, in which you work closely with the mentor (Hunt and Michael 1983). Following this a 'break up' is described, followed by lasting friendship (Hunt and Michael 1983). With short placements a common feature of nursing programmes, the extent to which either a break up or a lasting friendship occurs is uncertain. However, in a similar way to remembering your best teacher as a child, you will come across very good mentors, who will leave an impact on you and whom you may tend to remember long after your placement ends. Having a mentor in the clinical area can be extremely satisfying; indeed a 'mentorship relationship and a satisfied student go *hand in hand*' (Saarikoski *et al.* 2007). The only items that tend to negate against this satisfaction are practical ones, such as not having sufficient time scheduled to work together with the mentor or having an unavoidable change of mentor.

The portfolio can provide the medium for greater collaboration between you and your mentor, and even opening up the portfolio and going through it together opens up the communication channels and begins to build the relationship. This permits the mentor to ask you questions about your portfolio that prompts your further learning. It may be best to see the portfolio as a journey of discovery, upon which the mentor travels with you. Interestingly, from what we have learned so far in this book, there is nothing to suggest that you seek direction from the mentor in the first instance. In keeping with adult learning principles embedded in this whole approach, the first step begins with you.

Activity 3

In Activity 1 you identified mentor behaviours that assisted your learning.

Are your views consistent with any of the emerging attributes of facilitators?

Write down your views.

Working with your mentor to put the portfolio together

The mentor relationship, once developed, will be extremely helpful to you in terms of seeking guidance and support in relation to putting your portfolio together. Time needs to be set aside to be able to talk through your initial ideas with your mentor, and it might be worth arranging to set aside 15–20 minutes during the day for your first meeting. It is also important to do some thinking and preparation in advance of any scheduled meetings so that you have begun the learning process independently. From the perspective of both students (Lofmark and Wikblad 2001) and nursing staff, finding this time within the busyness of the clinical area can be difficult. However, you as a student can easily keep these meetings short, while maximizing their benefit, by thoroughly preparing in advance. This preparation includes taking along the folder, reading your guidelines in advance, and highlighting pertinent points. It is also useful to prepare your folder with the relevant dividers and outline some rough ideas for your learning needs and objectives. As the portfolio progresses the preparatory work will vary but it is important that it is completed.

Looking back at Chapter 6, the first phases of portfolio development are identified as follows:

1 Identify your own personal learning needs; document these in the portfolio.
2 Establish whether there are clear guidelines for your portfolio, and seek clarification if required. Use the guidelines to format the portfolio.
3 Once your broad learning needs have been identified these can be condensed and used as the basis for formulating objectives. Objectives are specific outcomes related to the portfolio; document these in the portfolio.

4 Using the guidelines or expected learning outcomes/activities, identify what it is you need to do to achieve the set goals. Use this to design or plan your learning experiences.
5 If your portfolio is linked to assessment of competence as described in Chapter 4, then you may need to attend the clinical placement, complete practice/competence documentation, engage with practice under the guidance of a facilitator/mentor, participate in holistic client care and gain exposure to a range of health care situations. You may also have specific personal learning needs based on your own previous experience.
6 Evaluate the process so far.
7 Select an approach to presentation (toast rack, spinal column or cake mix)*.
8 Select a model to underpin the overall approach.
9 Incorporate appropriate evidence within the model, using a series of entries.
10 Discuss and describe your entries and link them together.
11 Use a model of reflection, if appropriate, to develop entries.

The process begins with you identifying your learning needs and documenting these. This automatically reframes your relationship with your mentor, and requires you to approach the situation as an independent adult with some idea of your learning needs and to use these as the basis for a discussion with a view to sharing these with your mentor. If you have familiarized yourself with your learning requirements for the experience you ought to be able to identify your own needs. The mentor may be able to help you with appropriate wording, but the responsibility for putting these together will rest with you. These are personal to you, so there will be no right or wrong answers. You may at this point need to seek clarification on, and be guided by, your own local portfolio guidelines, which may have very specific requirements. If the portfolio contributes to summative assessment it is best to seek clarification from the person with overall responsibility for managing that assessment.

Your mentor's main role as facilitator of the portfolio is to assist you to achieve your goals. These will become clearer as you begin to outline your learning objectives. These too may be presented during the meetings in which you continue to share your thoughts and to seek the views of your mentor on the approach that you are taking. Again, it is very likely that you will have a fairly good idea of the objectives that you require, although how to word these appropriately may need to be further teased out with your mentor. Once confirmed, you can begin to plan your learning experiences in relation to your objectives. As your mentor is supporting your learning goals, there may be specific learning experiences that could be arranged in order for you to achieve specific objectives. Obviously a large proportion of the learning experiences

---

*Endacott *et al.* (2004) suggest four different ways of organizing your portfolio: the shopping trolley, the toast rack, the spinal column and the cake mix approaches. These are described in detail on pages 104–106.

that you describe will be suitably covered by simply attending your clinical placement, and specific details may not be required. However, if you have a particular need (perhaps you have not removed sutures yet for example), your mentor could work with you to provide maximum exposure to this experience, as appropriate.

If you are new to the clinical area it might be particularly difficult even to imagine the range of learning experiences that you could identify, and it has been suggested that junior students often require more mentor support than their more senior colleagues. An experienced mentor may be able to guide you towards competencies or objectives that are particularly suited to the area within which you are practising and about which you are likely to obtain substantial evidence. Once your plans are firmly in place, you may begin the task of simultaneously engaging the learning experiences and completing the portfolio.

Incorporating your learning experiences

The learning experiences that you have planned with your mentor and that you experience in your clinical practice may be linked to competencies or proficiency standards that are used to subdivide the folder (toast rack, spinal column), or subsection (cake mix), depending on the approach that you take. Obviously not all learning experiences will be documented, but perhaps with the assistance of your mentor you can pick out key learning experiences that may be described as an 'entry' to your portfolio. These can be described, and this will maintain the connecting dialogue that you require, but you also require suitable evidence to include with each entry. You may be encouraged, for example, to gain simple testimonies from staff related to a particular area of competence, or you may be encouraged to examine practice guidelines and discuss these. Other valuable learning experiences include observing the mentor during practical nursing experiences or taking part in these. The skill that has been observed or carried out can then be further elaborated by perhaps a description within the portfolio and a summary of a related research article. It could also be further expanded through reflection on the event, either contained as further evidence within the subsection (toast rack, spinal column) or contained within its own sub-theme (cake mix). As previously mentioned in Chapter 3, there is a tendency within reflections to focus on negative experiences, perhaps due to the use of the term 'incident' when ordinary events would suffice. The practice milieu exists as a learning experience and there are many opportunities to reflect upon day-to-day practice that will result in meaningful learning. Communicating with a patient is one example of an everyday skill that could be used. The section 'critical incident' within the cake mix approach could be substituted with 'reflections' to provide more appropriate guidance. Further types of evidence are now considered.

Gathering the evidence

Evidence in the portfolio is crucial; this helps to demonstrate the claims to learning that you are making (Jasper 2006). Portfolio entries do not stand alone but rather are supported by evidence (Jasper 2006) that are integrated carefully within the portfolio to demonstrate overall a cohesive logical approach. The task of mentors is not to police this operation, as freedom is paramount to the facilitation process. Students should be encouraged to think about inclusion items for a little time before brainstorming some ideas and then jotting them down. Mentors may act as a sounding board as students bounce ideas off them, but ultimately, through discussion, you as a student will be able to come to your own conclusions about what is the best evidence to provide. As the portfolio is a unique and individual construction there are no right or wrong answers in relation to inclusive evidence; however, making sense and having a logical flow to the work are important and must be borne in mind. There are practical limitations too in some cases; certain evidence may be too bulky to include and would therefore require a summary. When considering placing evidence within the portfolio, ask yourself why you are including it and what is its relevance and meaning. Simply including materials for the sake of it is of limited value in terms of learning to be achieved and leads you down the shopping trolley route. Placing a research article within, even if you have read it, doesn't explain to the reader where it fits in with either the specific section or the portfolio as a whole. Remember, those portfolios judged to be of greater merit in Endacott *et al.*'s (2004) study were those that maintained a continuous dialogue throughout the portfolio and brought readers step by step through the process. This dialogue doesn't have to be long and drawn out; it can simply be a brief summary and one or two lines of text to link one item to the next. Examples of evidence are provided in Box 7.1.

Box 7.1 Suggested evidence for inclusion within the portfolio

- Description of programme of reading (Price 2003): a brief list of references related to a topic, that are read and brief notes made on each.
- Description of practice project – key points on a practice-related project (Price 2003). Description of field trip or visit, including objectives and discussion of events (Price 2003). Description of observations from practice (Price 2003).
- Testimonies (Rassin *et al.* 2006).
- Competence documentation.
- Attendance records.
- Summaries of meetings with mentor.
- Summary of guidelines and protocols, or some aspect of these.

- Summary of patient information leaflets.
- Summary of research article related to practice.
- Summary of prior classroom learning on a topic.
- Videos or DVD of skills performed.
- Reflection.
- Case studies.

It is not suitable simply to include either primary or secondary evidence in the portfolio without appropriate discussion of their place within the portfolio (Jasper 2006). While your mentor cannot dictate the evolution of your portfolio, he or she can be helpful by reading through sections of the portfolio as it develops.

Using a model of reflection

The use of a model of reflection may or may not be a suggested dimension of your portfolio requirements. If it is to be included there may be some direction about where the reflection fits into the process. Learning from practice is an important facet of your educational programme, and reflection can serve to unlock some of this learning (Boud *et al.* 2006). Reflection may be presented as evidence within your portfolio, and in the absence of specific guidelines about choice of model, you may choose to select the model presented in Chapter 6 (Table 6.4). Within your discussion you may subdivide this process of reflection into critical analysis (where you examine policies, literature and other evidence); critical reflexivity (where you return to the experience, attend to your feelings, associate/integrate and validate these using appropriate information); and critical action (where you take action to improve your knowledge and skills base, and increase your awareness of the context within which your observations took place). An example of this model in use is provided in summary format below. However, you would obviously need to elaborate much more in each area in your portfolio, to include the relevant literature and support your reflections with dialogue. If you feel comfortable you may also share your unfolding reflections with your mentor.

Situation

During your clinical placement you have been trying to use touch with patients as much as possible. You believe that this is very helpful to patients, shows caring and reassures them. You pat people on the shoulder, or sometimes hold or rub their hands or rub their shoulders. One day a nurse calls you aside and suggests that this may not always be appropriate and that some patients may not like this. You are hurt by this comment and believe that this was said as an objection to you talking and showing care to patients. You include this within an entry in relation to the competence domain *Interpersonal relationships*.

Critical analysis

In your section on critical analysis you refer to ward policy (which is not explicit about the use of touch) and consult the literature on the topic. The literature indicates that, indeed, there are some groups of patients for whom a touch (albeit well intended) is not comfortable or welcome and patients can find the pat on the back or the head patronizing. Furthermore, you as a member of the health care team are in a powerful position in relation to touch, and have the ability to intervene in this way almost uninvited, where you wouldn't do so if you met the same person on the bus. While crossing this personal space through the use of touch can be beneficial and is encouraged within the nursing profession, there is limited research on how patients view this and negative patient views have been reported.

Critical reflexivity

From your previous critical analysis, you begin to engage yourself with the debate and question your own assumptions and values. Through your writing you return to the experience, attending to the feelings that you had with the event (embarrassment, hurt), but without dwelling on these, and you begin to associate the event with your understanding at that time (touch is common in your family and you are comfortable with this). You integrate your new information into your new understanding (the literature indicates that family experiences can influence how you perceive and use touch). You validate your new understandings (you begin to understand now that the touch you were demonstrating may not be in keeping with patient needs) and you appropriate this knowledge (make it your own). Through this you come to a negotiated understanding and take care to monitor your own behaviour against the standards and norms of the registered nurses with whom you work.

Critical action

- Your skill base in relation to the use of touch within nurse–patient communication and your awareness of the patients' perspective has increased.
- You decide to continue to read the research on this topic to inform your growing understanding and will also do a short presentation to the ward on your findings.
- Working alongside your mentor, you aim to inform ward policy and standards through your presentation.

Critical reflection is a key feature of facilitation (Rogers 1969, 1983). It is therefore important that the mentor guides you towards using reflection. Again, adequate training and preparation of the mentor is required so that the mentor may understand the process. However, the goal of the mentor here is not to teach you about reflection (that ought to happen in the classroom), or provide definitive direction about how to reflect, but rather perhaps to open a dialogue that is probing that might assist you to come up with ideas for reflection. The role of a mentor with regard to portfolio development is very much supportive of you in terms of listening and guiding (Hull *et al.* 2005).

Once a decision is reached to reflect upon a particular learning situation, you may be able to bounce ideas off the mentor in relation to the critical analysis that may proceed this reflexivity, and the mentor may indeed provide guidance as to whether you may access the relevant policies, or remind you to check through your classroom notes to see if pertinent information lies within. With regard to different level of analysis you may wish to summarize and describe local policy, for example, and also describe findings from an international literature perspective. The mentor may also provide confidence and encouragement for you to begin to write.

When *returning to the experience*, the mentor may support you by providing a quiet time for reflection and also remind you of the various components of the process. You may be tempted to cut past some aspects of a model of reflection, but it is important, particularly in relation to comprehensive evidence and validity of that evidence, that all processes are carried through. It is important that you, as a result of reflection, come to a new understanding about the situation, having perhaps questioned your own understanding of events. The critical analysis of knowledge assists in this new understanding. With regard to critical action, you, working alongside the mentor, may be able to make suggestions about practice issues that the nurse may present back to the area. Personal actions, such as improvements in particular skills, may also be an outcome of the critical practice framework for reflection, and thus the mentor may be in a position to facilitate this further required learning. Ultimately the action carried forward through both theoretical and personal reflection is an increased confidence and awareness around the subject under consideration.

The importance of the mentor relationship to reflection becomes obvious in the context of critical practice. As you develop from the process of reflection within the portfolio to becoming a critical practitioner, you will, through discussion with the mentor, come to new understandings about the practice. You may be concerned and embarrassed about showing reflective work to a mentor, and this is common. However, this may be due to the overly personal and ultimately self-development approach to other models of reflection that you may have used that are more suited to personal and private use (Jasper 2003). With the critical practice approach, the description and analysis is broader in terms of practice, and a mentor is important to facilitate your learning in this regard.

Farrell (2004) found that mentors' attitudes towards the students' use of reflection within their portfolio were positive. Most identified what they perceived to be the benefits of reflection for the students' development and for practice. It was noted, however, that some students appeared to procrastinate their reflection on practice, as they wanted to write 'a fantastic piece of work' or about an 'amazing event', so mentors urged 'all those involved within nurse education to reiterate the value of reflection on all aspects of care and not just the unusual or elitist events' (Farrell 2004: 79).

Your reflection may be facilitated while either attending the clinical practice area or within the classroom setting. It is important that you and your mentor take cognizance of the issues that surround reflection such as confidentiality, credibility and honesty. If your mentor facilitates your reflection there ought to be clear guidelines for a pathway for disclosure should you reveal items during reflective writing or discussions that may warrant reporting within the health service or elsewhere. These guidelines ought to be developed locally in a partnership arrangement with the Nursing School. Although it is beyond the remit of this book to consider all the practice issues that may arise as a result of student reflection, some brief guidelines in relation to ethical and legal issues are provided in Chapter 3.

Evaluation of your progress

It might be helpful for both mentor and student to read through the portfolio before final completion to examine the extent to which it is beginning to fulfil the criteria. Having an understanding of the marking criteria would help this process, and all parties would generally be aware of these in advance of port-folio completion. Using the marking criteria outlined in Chapter 2 as a guide, you could assess the standard of the content of your developing portfolio. Using the headings credibility, transferability, dependability, confirmability, adequateness and appropriateness of data and audit, for example, could lead to a useful discussion between you and your mentor about the standard that you have achieved. In relation to credibility, a mentor or student may question whether all data sources have been acknowledged. Is a reference list included and is it accurate? If a guideline from practice is used, is its origin and title clearly outlined? With regard to transferability, can the descriptions within the portfolio be applied in general to patients and to nursing practice? Or is it very anecdotal and personal and just one person's view of reality? Considering dependability, is the evidence authentic? When talking about confirmability, is a reader directed to the source of the evidence? Is it clear where the evidence is from? For example, if it relates to a research article, is a full reference pro-vided? It may be considered whether the evidence included is adequate or appropriate. Is there sufficient evidence to support the purported outcomes? Does it appear to be appropriate? Is there an obvious over-reliance on one type of knowledge, for example *phronesis* (practical and social wisdom – see Chapter 1) at the expense of other types of knowledge (e.g. empirical, research evidence)? This may weaken the portfolio impact. When considering audit, is there a comprehensive documentation of evidence to observe clearly how conclusions were drawn?

In addition, both you and your mentor may look at your emerging presentation of the portfolio. Does it fit together nicely in a cohesive way? Is the approach holistic and integrated? Or is it just a sum of its parts? Which approach would best describe it? With reference to the approaches to portfolio outlined in Chapter 5, does the portfolio reflect a shopping trolley approach or toast rack approach? Or is it blending together well, with either a spinal column or cake mix approach? At this point there is still time to reexamine both the content and the presentation in order to make the best of the information that is presented.

Conclusion

There are many ways in which you and your mentor can work together in this atmosphere of genuine mutual respect to achieve learning goals related to the portfolio. As facilitation and student-centred learning is at the core of this relationship, it is not expected necessarily that the mentor will directly and overtly teach you, but rather will encourage the student to learn for him or herself. This can be daunting for some students, particularly if they are used to a very directive teaching style from their own educational background. But it is important to remember, as a student, that this is a two-way relationship and that student effort is required. As the clinical learning environment experience is fundamentally about creating a bridge between what you have learned in the classroom and how this relates to practice, it may be expected, then, that from time to time you would refer back to your classroom learning and bring this information back into the clinical area through dialogue with your mentor, or perhaps through an entry in your portfolio. This is the means by which students become the active self-directed learner that the facilitation process requires (Burrows 1997). From the student's perspective, it is important that mentors take time to meet with students and look at the portfolio regularly and that they ask open and probing questions about the portfolio.

The continued development of formalized one-to-one supportive relationships for nursing students is advocated from an international perspective (Saarikoski et al. 2007). Supportive facilitative relationships within the health care environment can effectively support you in your development, particularly in relation to your portfolio. Mentors play a valuable role in facilitating the processes required for successful completion of the portfolio. In order to maximize the benefit of this relationship it is important that mentors are adequately prepared for their role in facilitation. It is important that they have an understanding of the processes required within the portfolio including reflection. Clear guidelines are also important. While ultimately the portfolio is a self-directed activity on behalf of the student, facilitation can motivate students towards achieving their goals in this area.

Summary of key points

- Mentors are key personnel in providing support and guidance for students undertaking portfolio development.
- Your mentor is not expected to provide explicit direction, but rather encourages you to be independent in your learning through providing support.
- Through entering into a professional relationship with your mentor, arranging a meeting and opening up a dialogue and discussion about your portfolio, you can both begin the voyage of discovery together.
- Important elements of the portfolio include: identifying learning needs; outlining objectives; identifying learning experiences; choosing a model and an approach to presentation; selecting the evidence and putting it all together in either toast rack, spinal column or cake mix approach.
- Dialogue and discussion are expected throughout the portfolio to tie subsections together. The final product ought to be connected in some way.

References

An Bord Altranais (2004) *Requirements and Standards for Nurse Registration* Education Programmes. Dublin: An Bord Altranais.

Andrews, M. and Wallis, M. (1999) Mentorship in nursing: a literature review, *Journal of Advanced Nursing*, 29(1): 201–7.

Boud, D., Cressey, P. *et al.* (2006) Setting the scene for productive reflection at work, D. Boud, P. Cressey and P. Doherty (eds) *Productive Reflection at Work*. Oxford: Routledge.

Burrows, D. E. (1997) Facilitation: a concept analysis, *Journal of Advanced Nursing*, 25(2): 396–404.

Cavanagh, S. J. and Snape, J. (1997) Education stress in student midwives: an occupational perspective, *British Journal of Midwifery*, 5(9): 528–33.

Endacott, R., Gray, M. A. *et al.* (2004) Using portfolios in the assessment of learning and competence: the impact of four models, *Nurse Education in Practice*, 4(4): 250–7.

Farrell, M. (2004) Illuminating the essential elements of the competence-based approach to nurse education through an exploration of staff nurses' experiences of its implementation within the practice placement: a phenomenological study. Masters Thesis, School of *Nursing and Midwifery*, University College Dublin.

Fulton, J., Bohler, A. *et al.* (2007) Mentorship: An international perspective, *Nurse Education in Practice*, 7(6): 399–406.

Hamill, C. (1995) The phenomenon of stress as perceived by project 2000 student nurses: a case study, *Journal of Advanced Nursing*, 21(3): 528–36.

Higgins, A. and McCarthy, M. (2005) Psychiatric nursing students' experiences of having a mentor during their first practice placement: an Irish perspective, *Nurse Education in Practice*, 5(4): 218–24.

Hull, C., Redfern, J. *et al.* (2005) *Profiles and Portfolios: A Guide for Health and Social Care*. Basingstoke: Palgrave Macmillan.

Hunt, D. M. and Michael, C. (1983) Mentorship: a career training and development tool, *The Academy of Management Review*, 8(3): 475–85.

Jasper, M. (2006) Portfolios and the use of evidence, in M. Jasper (ed.) *Professional Development, Reflection and Decision Making*, pp. 154–183, Oxford: Blackwell Publishing.

Jones, M. C. and Johnston, D. W. (2000) Reducing distress in first level and student nurses: a review of the applied stress management literature, *Journal of Advanced Nursing*, 32(1): 66–74.

Lambert, V. and Glacken, M. (2004) Clinical support roles: a review of the literature, *Nurse Education in Practice*, 4(3): 177–83.

Lindop, E. (1999) A comparative study of stress between pre- and post-Project 2000 students, *Journal of Advanced Nursing*, 29(4): 967 73.

Lofmark, A. and Wikblad, K. (2001) Facilitating and obstructing factors for development of learning in clinical practice: a student perspective, *Journal of Advanced Nursing*, 34(1): 43–50.

Mahat, G. (1996) Stress and coping: first year Nepalese nursing students in clinical settings. *Journal of Nursing Education*, 35(4): 163–9.

May, K. M., Meleis, A. I. *et al.* (1982) Mentorship for scholarliness: opportunities and dilemmas, *Nursing Outlook*, 30(1): 22–8.

O'Donovan, M. (2006) Reflecting during clinical placement – discovering factors that influence pre-registration psychiatric nursing students, *Nurse Education in Practice*, 6(3): 134–40.

Pearce, R. (2003) *Profiles and Portfolios of Evidence*. Cheltenham: Nelson Thornes.

Rhead, M. H. (1995) Stress among student nurses: is it practical or academic?, *Journal of Clinical Nursing*, 4(6): 369–76.

Rogers, C. R. (1969) *Freedom to Learn*, Princeton, NC: Merrill.

Rogers, C. R. (1983) *Freedom to Learn for the 80s*, Princeton, NC: CE Merrill Publishing Company.

Saarikoski, M., Marrow, C. *et al.* (2007) Student nurses' experience of supervision and mentorship in clinical practice: a cross-cultural perspective, *Nurse Education in Practice*, 7(6): 407–15.

Thyer, S. E. and Bazeley, P. (1993) Stressors to student nurses beginning tertiary education: an Australian study, *Nurse Education Today*, 13(5): 336–42.

Index

THE PRESCRIPTION DRUG GUIDE FOR NURSES

Sue Jordan

This book is exceedingly timely. I am certain it will be invaluable to both undergraduate and post graduate student nurses, and, also act as a continuing reference source. Thoroughly recommended.

Molly Courtenay, Reading University, UK

Sue Jordan has combined her deep understanding of her own discipline with her long experience of teaching nurses, to produce just the right type and level of information that nurses need, in a format that they will find relevant to their practice and easy to use. This book will be an essential reference resource for every ward bookshelf.

Professor Dame June Clark, Swansea University, UK

This popular *Nursing Standard* prescription drug series is now available for the first time in book format! Organised by drug type and presented in an easy-to-use reference format, this book outlines the implications for practice of 20 drug groups.

Each drug group is presented in handy quick check format, and covers:

- Drug actions
- Indications
- Administration
- Adverse effects
- Practice suggestions
- Cautions/contra-indications
- Interactions

Contents

Preface – Using this book – Abbreviations used in the text – Introduction – Laxatives – Controlling gastric acidity – Diuretics – Beta blockers – ACE inhibitors – Vasodilators (calcium channel blockers and nitrates) – Anticoagulants – Bronchodilators: Selective beta2 adrenoreceptor agonists – Corticosteroids – Antipsychotics – Antidepressants: Focus on SSRIs – Anti-emetics – Opioid analgesics – Anti-epileptic drugs: Focus on carbamazepine and valproate – Antibacterial drugs – Insulin – Oral anti-diabetic drugs – Thyroid and anti-thyroid drugs – Cytotoxic drugs – Non-steroidal anti-inflammatory drugs (NSAIDs) – Idiosyncratic drug reactions – Glossary – References – Bibliography/ Further Reading – Index.

March 2008   192pp
978–0–335–22547–7 (Paperback)   978–0–335–22546–0 (Hardback)

SURVIVING YOUR PLACEMENT IN HEALTH AND SOCIAL CARE
A STUDENT HANDBOOK

Joan Healey and Margaret Spencer

This attractive workbook provides a wealth of tools and 'top tips' for students of health and social care struggling to survive the demands of 21st century practice placements. The authors artfully distil their knowledge, experience and expertise in placement learning in order to accompany the student on their journey from novice to qualified professional.
Stephanie Hobson, Head of Practice Education, Oxford Brookes University, UK

I found the text to be set at a good level for new students of nursing, allied health and social care especially for the early placements in their programme of study. In an easy and engaging style the book offer a range of useful tools to helps students make the most and get the best from their placement experiences. I would be happy to recommend this to students on a range of courses.
George Bell, Northumbria University, UK

As students in health and social care professions, you will spend up to half of your time out on placement. This accessible and practical book is designed to help you make the most of this invaluable learning experience and is suitable for use in all areas of practice, whether you are training to be a nurse, midwife, occupational therapist, social worker or physiotherapist.

In student friendly language it covers all the main areas of placement learning, including:

- Developing a learning contract
- Reflective practice
- Using supervision
- Managing time
- Evidence-based practice
- Capturing your learning in a personal and professional portfolio
- Failing placements

This book of highly practical chapters provides reflection exercises, questions, tests, ideas and tools to use on your placement, case studies to read and practical tips throughout to help you achieve your best on placement, in whatever area of practice you are in.

Surviving Your Placement in Health and Social Care is key reading for all health and social care students, including nurses, social workers, physiotherapists, occupational therapists and radiographers amongst other.

Contents
Using this book – Preparing yourself for placement – Reflective practice – Writing learning objectives – Assessment – Complex decision making and professional reasoning – Balance and time management – Supervision – The personal and professional development process – Interprofessional perspectives on placement – Evidence based practice and using the internet – Failure – Not quite the end . . .

2007   176pp

978–0–335–22259–9 (Paperback)   978–0–335–22260–5 (Hardback)

ESSENTIAL CALCULATION SKILLS FOR NURSES AND MIDWIVES

Meriel Hutton

Calculation skills are a core part of nursing and midwifery practice, from calculating drug or medicine doses to monitoring a patients' liquid intake or stock management. It is also an area for concern, as evidence shows that both qualified nurses and trainee students are seriously lacking in basic numeracy skills.

This key book provides a guide to calculation skills and includes the core charts, prescription models, labels and diagrams (such as syringes) needed by student and practising nurses or midwifes.

Importantly this text will provide context through the use of senarios and examples that refer to all branches of nursing and midwifery.

Contents
Basic mathematical skills – Fluid balance charts – Medications safety – Oral medications – Injections and IV fluids – More complex calculations for critical care areas.

December 2008 152pp

978–0–335–23359–5 (Paperback)

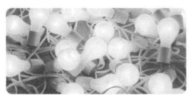
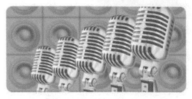
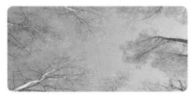
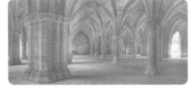
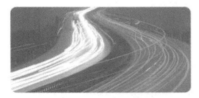
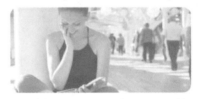
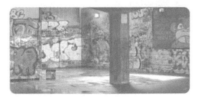